TRICARE: Betrayal In The Philippines Is This the Future of TRICARE Overseas?

James B. Houtsma

Foreward by David Paraiso

David Paraiso
2013

First Printing: 2013

ISBN 978-0-9907625-3-9

David Paraiso

Foreword by David Paraiso

We thank Jim for sharing the tragic experience of Tricare beneficiaries in the Philippines. Being imbedded within the system for several decades and with his meticulous documentation of the pertinent chain of events and specific cases, this book describes the DHA/TMA and ISOS bureaucracy running amuck and in self-denial in the Philippines and which, among other things, could be perpetuating this tragedy from country to country. After many years of assisting and advocating in behalf of Tricare beneficiaries, and with no substantive response from the bureaucracy - this book is the last resort for Jim.

Who are the primary victims here? Reply: Tricare beneficiaries and the U.S. taxpayers (represented by the U.S. Congress).

The description of the book summarizes Jim's major findings. Jim may be contacted at ForgottenFewPI@gmail.com.

Jim was originally from Chico, CA. He was with the U.S. Army from 1963 thru 1983. He was honorably discharged and retired with a rank of 1SG on April 1, 1983.

He went back to work in civil service and between May 1984 thru March 2004, Jim performed a variety of assignments as Chief, Mgmt BR, RMD, Health System Analyst, in Operations Management, and Director DSS Support at the following organizations, Raymond W. Bliss Army Community Hospital, Ft. Huachuca, AZ, Patient Administration Systems and Biostatistics Activity (PASBA), Ft. Sam Houston, TX, Mental Health Care Line (MHCL), Southern AZ VA Health Care System, Tucson, AZ, and Business Service Line, Management Support, Southern AZ VA Health Care System, Tucson, AZ.

Jim moved to the Philippines in March 2004.

Since February 2005, Jim has been a volunteer assisting TRICARE Beneficiaries in the Philippines. He started a Yahoo forum to support the military retirees spread out in hundreds of islands.

Jim was a recipient of the following:
1. Meritorious Service Medal (First Oak Leaf Cluster), 1983

2. Meritorious Service Medal, 1980

3. Army Commendation Medal (First Oak Leaf Cluster), 1971

4. Army Commendation Medal, 1968

5. Commendation from the Army Surgeon General in 1998 and 1999

6. Commanders Award for Civilian Service, 1990, 1992 and 1999

7. Achievement Medal for Civilian Service, 1993 and again in 1996

Other accomplishments:
1. Participated in the publishing of a paper on the Evaluation of Ambulatory Care Classification Systems for the Military Health Care System, 1990

2. Co-authored "Establishing the Environment for Implementation of a Data Quality Management Culture in the Military Health System" (1998). Paper presented at the 1998 Conference on Information Quality, Massachusetts Institute of Technology

3. Co-authored "Establishing an Operational Data Quality Practice" (1999). Paper presented at the 1999 Conference on Information quality, Massachusetts Institute of Technology

4. Presented "Datascan Alternatives in MEPRS" at the Army Surgeon General's worldwide MEPRS conference, 1988

5. Presented "Cost Reduction through Physician Profiling and Clinic Level Budgets" at the Southwest Federal Health Care Consortium Meeting, 1992

6. Presented "Concepts and Tools for a Successful Clinically Driven Utilization Management Program" (Co-presented with LTC Jill Phillips) and "How to Get the Data You Need" at Health Services Command's Ambulatory Care Conference, 1993

7. Presented "Successful Integration of Health Promotion, Utilization and Cost Savings into a Clinically Driven Managed Care Program" and "The Price of Doing Business Right...and Wrong" (both Co-presented with LTC Jill Phillips) at Health Services Command's TRICARE Conference, Jan. 1994

8. Coordinated six separate two-day PASBA regional Data Quality Symposiums and conducted five hours of presentations on data quality issues at each symposium. These symposiums trained over 1,400 MHS staff at over 100 facilities on the importance of data quality in health care automated systems, 1996 to 1999

9. Was a principle presenter at a three-day VISN 18 and 21 DSS workshop, 2002

10. In 1994 independently developed a methodology to convert Defense Eligibility Enrollment Reporting System (DEERS) demographic data into a format that would be accepted by the Composite Health Care System (CHCS)

Background

I moved to the Philippines in early 2004. Because of my background in health care administration and TRICARE and because TRICARE was my medical insurance plan I had a particular interest in how it operated in the Philippines and how it was perceived by beneficiaries and local health care professionals. I soon found there was no formal information on the already modified program. There were the normal standard descriptions but nothing about the growing and significant modifications that applied to Philippine TRICARE. The military retirees I spoke to had little understanding either. It was also obvious to me many had some misunderstandings of the program.

There are no military bases and so no Health Benefits Advisors (HBA) in the Philippines. So I tried to contact the closest HBA which was in Guam. I went to the TRICARE webpage where there was a list of HBA's worldwide with email addresses. I sent an email to the HBA in Guam but it was ignored. I sent a second email and it was also ignored. So I contacted a retired Army LTC I knew who worked in Washington D.C., explained the problem and asked if he knew someone at the TRICARE Management Activity (TMA) that I might contact who could provide information or direct me to someone that did. He gave me the email address of an Army Col, ANC, who worked there. I emailed her but she was irritated that I contacted her and told me to contact my local HBA. I explained to her we had no local HBAs and my attempt to contact one in Guam was ignored. Her response was, "Then contact another one." So I obtained all the email addresses of all the HBAs on the Pacific Rim but outside the U.S. and sent them an email explaining the problem and the lack of a response from Guam. A third came back as invalid email addresses. Of the balance an HBA in Japan responded saying he knew the rules were different for the Philippines but didn't know what they were and suggested I talk to other retirees in the Philippines as he knew of no source for the information. Another individual contacted me saying she had not been an HBA for a year but suggested I contact an individual in Hawaii and provided the email address. The individual in Hawaii also said she knew little about the differences and suggested I contact an Air Force LTC who was on the way to Okinawa to help open a TRICARE Area Office for the Pacific. I contacted him but he said he was in transit and to give him a couple of months to get there and set up.

At the time I lived in Bicol in southern Luzon so thought maybe by contacting other military retirees in other areas they might know more as I was having little success. I started a Yahoo forum in 2005 for military retirees living in the Philippines in the hope of finding others with more knowledge and also as a way to educate others about their medical benefit in the Philippines. I discovered, based on that input that there was a requirement to use what was called "Certified" providers. Most had no idea how to determine who was certified and who was not but one individual provided a web address to a Naval hospital on Okinawa where there was supposed to be a list. However he cautioned that the list seemed to change by the month and names of providers would appear one month but then disappear the next month. Over a period of months as more joined the group we found people that had used providers that appeared on the list but had their claims denied because the provider was not certified. Others claimed they used providers who were not on the list but their claims were paid.

Ultimately and with the help of the staff at the new TRICARE Area Office – Pacific (TAO-P) we determined that the posted list was nothing more than a list of names from a month's worth of communications between International SOS (ISOS)[1] and Wisconsin Physician Services (WPS) and had no relationship to who was a certified provider. The file was provided by ISOS and my first indication of the quality of their work.

This was my first introduction to TRICARE in the Philippines. Years of working with military retirees and their family members from all over the Philippines, including assisting with claims, has

---

[1] ISOS created a local company known as Global 24 Network Services in 2012. They were presented to TMA and us as a local company with a history of developing medical networks. I became suspicious when there was no evidence of this company on the internet. But a month later a webpage appeared. What was troubling was major players at ISOS were prominently displayed on the page. Further investigation showed that the page was really the property of ISOS in Singapore and rented from Godaddy in the U.S. While we were told they would provide local phone and email support to Demo beneficiaries we also found that in truth we were calling ISOS in Singapore and the same people that man the ISOS help desk were also supposed to be working for Global 24; initially they would answer the phone as ISOS when we called the Global 24 number. Further we found that this company has no local physical address. Because of this when we refer to ISOS we may also be referring to Global 24.

2

given me a fairly good prospective on how they perceive the TRICARE benefit in the Philippines.

During this time I also joined a Rotary group in my area which included a number of physicians. Through this association I also met and interacted with hospital administrators. I learned a lot about how the local health care industry operates and the differences from the U.S. system. I also gained, from those that had TRICARE patients, their prospective on TRICARE. These interactions with health care professionals and beneficiaries continued as I moved to different locations within the Philippines.

Starting in 2005 I had interaction with multiple TMA staff at TAO-P, in Aurora CO and Washington D.C. which included discussions with the Deputy Director of TMA, MG Granger, who I previously worked with and kept in contact with for more than 20 years. I also communicated with some of the staff I knew from years before when we worked together on various projects. The senior civilian staff at TMA objected to these discussions and eventually was able to terminate most of them once MG Granger retired. I also had telephone and email discussions with the Lead Investigator for TRICARE fraud in the Philippines from the Defense Criminal Investigative Service (DCIS). He said he spent close to a year in the Philippines investigation fraud and his prospective of fraud here was significantly different from the prospective I encountered from many TMA employees, most of whom never visited the Philippines.

These discussions and interactions with these divergent groups who were all involved in different ways with TRICARE in the Philippines is the basis for the information to follow. I maintained virtually all emails and other relevant documents from 2005 to present. I've tried to relate times, places and circumstances to the best of my ability based on memory and these documents.

In early to mid-2011 two of us put together an extensive packet of documents showing the actions and results of TMA actions in the Philippines as well as contractor failures to comply with their contract and fraud on the part of the contractor. We also showed where we had made clear attempts to let TMA know of the consequences of their actions and the failures and fraud on the part of their contractor. Included were examples of beneficiary hardship as well. We contacted various attorney groups attempting to find one that would agree to take on these issues in a class action suit. We found one such group in California who spent months reviewing our information including Skype conferences and confirming the existence of documents in the possession of TMA that an informant claimed were there, increasing his credibility. While they said they felt we had a solid case that could be won, they said because of the small base of beneficiaries there would not be sufficient revenue for them to carry it forward. We offered to agree to donate any awards that beneficiaries might be granted as well but they said that was against the law. They advised us to go public with our information to try to force the government to correct the wrongs. Our attempts to find media willing to produce material was not successful. One reporter said that because we were overseas and half way around the world from the United States, an article would garner little interest there.

Others, primarily in the Yahoo forum, have contributed effort to understand and correct these wrongs. Writing this book is another attempt to get our story told.

Hyperlinks were removed and replaced with italics and associated endnotes.

What is TRICARE

TRICARE is a medical care plan for the Department of Defense Military Health System. It provides health benefits for military personnel, military retirees, and their dependents from the private health care industry.

In 1967 a medical benefit program called CHAMPUS was created by Congress. The Military Medical Benefits Amendments of 1966, Pub. L. No. 89-614, § 3, 80 Stat. 862, 866 (1966) brought retirees, their family members and certain surviving family members of deceased military sponsors into CHAMPUS.

In 1993 the program was renamed "TRICARE" and introduced three options; TRICARE Prime, TRICARE Standard and TRICARE Extra. (CHAMPUS evolved into TRICARE Standard) and the program was extended overseas.

Like a typical medical insurance plan it should, at a minimum, provide:

- Quality Care
- Choice of providers
- Good access to care
- Easy reimbursement for covered medical bills

We will find, wither compared to TRICARE in other countries or private insurance, none of these expectations are not being met in the Philippines.

TRICARE in the Philippines

The Philippines has the second largest population of TRICARE Standard beneficiaries of any country outside the United States as reported by the *DOD Office of the Actuary*[i]. This population, contrary to claims by the Department of Defense Inspector General (DODIG) and TMA/DHA[2] has slowly but steadily increased since TRICARE was implemented overseas.

Of the top six countries with populations of over 1,000 military retirees, the Philippines is the only one with no military bases and the accompanying TRICARE support such as Health Benefits Advisors (HBA). This also means there is no on the ground military medical staff who can provide feedback to TMA/DHA on issues of quality of care, access to care, local health care industry culture and issues with processing of claims.

When TRICARE Overseas was implemented the plan and rules in the Philippines were identical to all other countries. However, as we will see and in part due to the isolation addressed above, it wasn't long before that started to change. These changes had profound and far reaching consequences; including creating an environment that was conducive to fraud.

The Early Years

In 1991 Mount Pinatubo erupted. It was the second largest volcanic eruption of the 20th century. This and a growing resentment by Filipinos to the large military presence resulted in the closure of all bases and the removal of military personnel. The large contingent of retired military, their families and widows were left to fend for themselves. There was no program to provide medical care so those that could afford it paid for their own care while others did without.

Around the 1995 time frame the TRICARE Overseas Program (TOP) began in earnest. Beneficiaries in the Philippines were isolated

---

[2] In 1996 a government organization known as the TRICARE Management Activity (TMA) was responsible for the management of the program. They had offices in Falls Church, VA and Aurora, CO. In the early 2000's they added three overseas regional offices known as "TRICARE Area Offices". In October 2013 it was consolidated under the umbrella of the Defense Health Agency (DHA). From this point on we will refer to these entities as TMA/DHA.

from the infrastructure available to other large populations of Standard beneficiaries overseas and the population had begun to disperse from the traditional areas around the old base locations since there was little to hold them there; a trend that continues to grow as the years pass. In addition hundreds of Filipino-Americans who retired from the U.S. military had returned to enjoy their retirement in the Philippines and chose to live in the region from where they originally came. Because of the lack of infrastructure and the disbursement of the affected population, the second largest overseas population of TRICARE Standard beneficiaries lacked information on the new program. Many of those that heard about it lacked information on what was covered or how and where to file claims. Slowly and mostly around the two old military bases information got out. But for a significant portion of the population outside these areas they knew nothing of the benefit.

The First Fraud

Shortly after this a small group of Filipino-American military retirees near one of the bases were caught filing false claims for medical care and hospitalizations for themselves and their families. They were subsequently *convicted*[ii] for these crimes. The crime involved filing claims using the names of real or fake providers and could have been accomplished in any country in the same fashion. TMA/DHA reacted quickly by implementing the first of many policies that applied only to the Philippines and hired a contractor, ISOS, to implement the new "Certified provider" requirement but failed to inform the majority of beneficiaries of the changes or provide a viable list of certified providers.

Now the stage was set for someone to take advantage of these shortfalls. In other words provide access to care to those that found they could no longer see providers and get reimbursed for the care and those that had no information on the new TRICARE Overseas Program (TOP) or how to file claims.

Health Visions Corp. Comes on the Scene

At the time close to 100% of beneficiary claims were being denied due to the certified provider requirement. An individual felt he could provide a service by assisting. So he opened a clinic, Health

Visions Corp. (HVC), where he promised to obtain care for TRICARE beneficiaries and process their claims. The initial concept was good and designed to facilitate access to care. But early on greed took front seat. HVC learned how provider certification worked and formed a close relationship with ISOS who willingly certified providers they wanted to use, paying most of them at the local rates and then billing TMA/DHA at U.S. rates. In addition they offered, for a small premium, a policy that would cover the deductible and co-pays.[3] HVC started in Olongapo, an area with a large retiree population and it wasn't long before everyone was flocking to the clinic. Why? Because they now had a place to go and get medical care without the hassle of filing claims and better still without having most claims denied and having to pay the full cost of care themselves due to the unique and mostly unpublicized change in the TRICARE program; a poorly implemented and publicized change that required the use of only certified providers and applied only to the Philippines.

For reasons I never fully understood TMA/DHA chose to ignore the HVC fraud. I was told they were not prepared to deal with fraud since it was not part of their mandate when managing TRICARE in the states. They even resisted suggestions by the Defense Criminal Investigative Service (DCIS) and the DODIG to implement administrative measures already at their disposal to curb the growing fraud. For almost ten years HVC was allowed to grow and prosper as it expanded across the Philippines seeking out beneficiaries that TMA/DHA was never aware existed. This *map*[iii] shows how large this group became and also demonstrates the approximate distribution of beneficiaries across the Philippines. This failure on the part of TMA/DHA not only cost the taxpayer but set the stage for future fraud and resentment of TRICARE by providers. Between TMA/DHA and their contractor's actions provider fraud continued. Some deliberately and some due to contractor involvement that

---

[3] TMA/DHA claimed for years that beneficiaries should have known that this offer was not valid, not properly licensed within the Philippines and that the premiums were too low. While someone like myself might ascertain this, the average retiree and in particular their Filipino born wife would have no idea what would constitute a valid premium that could sustain such a policy and with a professional looking pamphlet to go along with the promotion it looked legitimate to the majority. This is one of the stereotypes that TMA/DHA has of retirees living in the Philippines; one that sees all retirees as intent on defrauding TRICARE for as much as possible.

8

caused many to believe what they were doing was legitimate and expected.

Finally caving in to pressure from the DCIS, DODIG and Congress, starting in 2006 TMA/DHA started to implement various new restrictions on the now totally unique TRICARE Philippine Standard.

The first act was to secretly stop payment on claims to most hospitals in the Philippines which was implemented on 8 November 2006; the claims contractor was instructed not to tell beneficiaries why their claims were not being processed. The freeze included both beneficiary and provider submitted claims. TMA/DHA Program Integrity wrongly believed that all these hospitals were directly involved in the HVC fraud and benefited from it which was not true and showed how little they really understood about the fraud. MG Granger was concerned how this secret freeze would affect beneficiaries who filed claims and was told by his staff that only a very few would be affected. That was absolutely untrue and on 17 March 2007 when I discovered what was going on I emailed him with a long email explaining the process of how they paid for the care at local rates and submitted inflated claims using their address to receive the check. Once he discovered how much harm was being done the freeze was lifted within days of my email on all hospitals except those owned by HVC.

The TMA/DHA Modifications to the Philippine Benefit

Certification of Providers

The first modification to TRICARE Overseas Standard was adding a requirement to use "Certified Providers". It was not well thought out and had dire consequences for the taxpayer and beneficiaries alike.

An assumption apparently was made that this fraud by military retirees living overseas couldn't occur anywhere else in the world but the Philippines, so the solution was only applied to the Philippines. Not that the conditions weren't available in other countries but that military retirees living elsewhere apparently would never do this. One might have also assumed that it was an isolated incident and not related to being a retiree in the Philippines as well but that wasn't the conclusion. So a system to certify providers as legitimate providers was instituted. The solution costs TMA/DHA hundreds of thousands of dollars a year to implement. Even more was lost to fraud this policy drove in conjunction with their contractor. This cost has gone on for more than fifteen years; most would not consider that as a cost effective solution in and of itself.

The reality is that this process would not stop the same kind or similar fraud from happing again if someone decided to do it. All someone has to do is have receipts printed using the name and address of a provider on the certified list and proceed in the same way by filing claims using the fake receipts. So in essence all the loss of access to care and the hundreds of thousands of dollars in denied claims, as detailed below, accomplished nothing of real value.

The real cost to TMA/DHA was yet to come however. When they implemented the certified provider list and required beneficiaries to use them in order to be paid, they failed to properly inform beneficiaries and failed to provide a valid list of providers that were certified. All the beneficiary knew was they their claim was denied and they were stuck with the cost. Further there was no office available that could assist these beneficiaries.

Even if they discovered the "official" list of certified providers that was buried on the web page of a Navy Hospital in Japan; it was not a true list of certified providers. In fact it was nothing more than a list created from the monthly summary of provider information that was transmitted between ISOS and Wisconsin Physician Services (WPS). In reality it was a list of provider names that were pending certification, denied certification or removed from the list for various reasons. Therefore providers that were certified in the past didn't show on the list and names disappeared after a month. The odds were if someone actually used a provider on the list they would find that the provider was not certified and their claim denied. So beneficiaries, even if they used the list, found their claims denied and there was nobody they could contact about the denial as there was nobody in the Philippines or anywhere else with the responsibility to assist beneficiaries; The TRICARE Area Office – Pacific (TAO-P) didn't exist until years later and has also proven to be of little benefit to beneficiaries. More and more beneficiaries found that their claims were denied and they had no idea why except they knew they were stuck with the cost of their care. This was a true failure on TMA/DHA's part to inform beneficiaries of drastic and unprecedented changes in their benefit and the catalyst that assisted fraud to get a foothold and lead to an unprecedented loss of access to care as well as tens of millions of dollars in excessive cost to taxpayers.

Beneficiaries were seeing providers, submitting claims, and hoping that they would get paid only to discover that the claim was denied because the provider was not certified. What they didn't know because TMA/DHA never told them, was that once they submitted a claim and it was denied, the provider would be scheduled for certification and once that was accomplished they could resubmit their claim. Instead they received a cryptic note saying, "Denied, Provider not certified". Even if they knew that they could resubmit the claim there was no way to determine if the provider was ever certified or denied certification due to the lack of a list; later we learned that beneficiaries were not to know the outcome of certification either. A growing number of beneficiaries were finding that their medical benefit was no longer available to them and paying for their own care. They were promised a medical benefit by Congress but then found it didn't work.

In addition there is an unpublicized policy that once a provider declined to be certified ISOS would inform WPS the provider was not certified and all future claims filed where that provider was used were denied. Beneficiaries had no way of knowing who had declined certification, because it was kept secret, so they had to take their chances. A review of seven years of the certified provider database showed that, on average, more than 100 providers declined certification a year. So after fifteen years there were more than a 1,500 providers that would never be certified but beneficiaries are not allowed to know who they were. One can only guess how many thousands of claims have been denied for care with legitimate licensed providers due to this policy alone.

Years later after I arrived and discovered the truth about the certified list it was finally fixed, at least to some extent. The revised list put out by TAO-P used data supplied by ISOS which was and still is fraught with errors and omissions. The list failed to provide basic information expected from such a list such as specialty, phone number and in many cases an actual address. Providers where listed with wrong cities, names misspelled and more. Appeals to TMA/DHA to improve the quality of the list were ignored with a comment that the quality of the list was "adequate" for beneficiaries in the Philippines. Over an 8 year period I and some others were able to publish examples of the horrible data on the internet and push TMA/DHA to require the contractor make some modest improvements. But the quality of the list is far from the standards seen by Active Duty around the world and all beneficiaries in the U.S.

Health Visions Corp. Allowed to Prosper

The original, faulty certified list was one of the catalysts that aided in the success of HVC and their fraudulent schemes.

Where TMA/DHA failed in their mandate to provide access to care and keep beneficiaries informed of their benefit, HVC appeared to keep that promise so it became a success over night. They also advertised that they were TRICARE's official sanctioned representative in the Philippines and TMA/DHA failed to ever refute that claim to beneficiaries or providers from which they purchased care.[4]

HVC opened its doors in 1998 and early on some retirees suspected that there was fraud involved and reported it. But, as has proven typical, TMA/DHA failed to provide any feedback to those that made the reports and also took no visible action. In fact, as we now know, they didn't take any action. Nor did they even attempt to counter claims by this organization that they were the "official" and "sanctioned" TRICARE provider in the Philippines. Since claims were always paid and years went by without a word out of TMA/DHA, local retirees began to believe the hype and even those that initially reported suspected fraud, as early as 1998, had to admit that it must be okay since TMA/DHA was doing nothing to stop the clinic and always paid the claims unlike claims filed by beneficiaries.[5]

---

[4] Over time HVC developed a relationship with many doctors, hospitals and others, claiming to be the official representative of TRICARE and using that claim to obtain credit with these providers. When HVC closed its doors it left tens of thousands of dollars owed too many of these providers and, to this day, they blame not HVC but TRICARE and the U.S. government for reneging on their obligations. This was a topic of discussion at Philippine Hospital Association meetings and one of the reasons why many hospitals will not consider filing claims for reimbursement and why providers decline certification.

[5] Because I worked with the health care system and TMA/DHA in the past I was aware that they tended to take years to do what should be done in months so suspected that sooner or later there would be repercussions but the average retiree that had not worked in the military health care field had no way of knowing that and believed the propaganda. In addition when claims always seemed to be paid when filed by HVC but often denied with little usable explanation when beneficiaries filed them it didn't take long before the average

As the years went by the clinic grew into a large company and expanded to every location in the Philippines where there were pockets of beneficiaries and this continued expansion further convinced beneficiaries that they were what they claimed to be since TMA/DHA remained silent. In fact HVC found retirees that knew nothing of the benefit, since they had retired before it was available, and apprised them of their benefit, in essence doing TMA/DHA's job of keeping beneficiaries informed of their medical benefit.[6]

Almost ten years would pass before TMA/DHA took any action and even then only due to extensive pressure from Congress and the DODIG who hit the nail on the head when they said in their report that TMA/DHA and WPS were negligent in allowing known fraud to continue for years. In their defense the office was not previously involved with fraud in the states as it was turned over to other agencies. Nor did they have staff or training to handle fraud on their own. But there were actions they could have taken if they had wanted.

So, let me ask you, who should take primary responsibility for the fraud in the Philippines? Instead of taking their lumps for neglecting to do their job, TMA/DHA decided to make things harder on the beneficiaries as they saw them as the root of all their problems. After all if they hadn't used HVC for care there would never have been a problem for TMA/DHA.[7]

Let's review. When TMA/DHA initiated the certified provider list without proper thought, publicity and follow through, they set the stage for the defrauder by driving beneficiaries that simply wanted to

---

beneficiary believed that TMA/DHA wanted them to use HVC, if not by word by actions.

[6] The TRICARE Overseas Program was relatively new and many retired military Filipino-Americans and others who retired and moved to the Philippines knew nothing of the program. They had assimilated into Philippine society and no real effort was made to inform them of the new benefit. So, even today, their knowledge of the program is what they were told by HVC who claimed to be the official representative of TRICARE. So to these people any group that looks and feels like HVC is TRICARE. The promised local office would have gone a long way in changing this belief.

[7] I was told by TMA/DHA employees we are all a bunch of lazy old men who live the good life of luxury in mansions with multiple maids, drivers and gardeners but were not satisfied with what we had so we devise ways to defraud TRICARE. Even when I was trying to work with them and addressed the lack of specialty and phone numbers and consistent addresses on the certified provider list I was told that the list was "adequate" for retirees in the Philippines. In essence we didn't deserve what others have and they didn't see a need to go the extra mile for us because of these perceptions which dehumanized us making it easier for them to ignore the suffering. I believe this stereotyping has been a contributing factor to the fraud and loss of access to care since they don't believe we deserve anything more than "adequate".

receive their benefit towards them. When they were forced to act, or maybe a better term would be react, they blamed the beneficiary for all their problems even convincing Congress that beneficiaries were heavily involved in the fraud and deserved what they got. The truth was while a few actively participated in fraud the majority did not. The way the certified list was implemented and maintained by the contractor and without any supervision from TMA/DHA allowed for it to be used as vehicle for more fraud; fraud that TMA/DHA would also see as the fault of beneficiaries.

Workgroup Formed to Identify Ways to Eliminate Fraud

Under pressure from DCIS, DODIG and Congress TMA/DHA was forced to react. Almost ten years had passed and the HVC fraud had grown to include most of the Philippines and new copycat operations were now in the mix as well. Groups such as Western Pacific Medical Services, Inc. A workgroup was formed to identify ways to reduce fraud. Most of the policy changes suggested by TMA/DHA were poorly designed and in addition to reducing fraud, they hurt beneficiaries by making obtaining care and getting reimbursed even more difficult than before. With no staff on the ground who would understand the differences in the local health care system and culture, many of these changes were programmed to fail or be used against TMA/DHA. Many also limited access to care and denied payment of legitimate claims which may have been unknown to the decision makers at TMA/DHA. The end result of these policies, along with their contractor, continued to drive fraud and a significantly reduced medical benefit for beneficiaries. This premise is further made when one considers that the one policy change that all those outside TMA/DHA, who were part of the workgroup, recommended would have actually reduced fraud the most and would also have increased access to care. Those from outside voiced concern to TMA/DHA that their changes would increasingly limit access to care but the locally contracted PPO suggestion was junked in favor of the TMA/DHA changes.[8]

The above is reinforced when reading an *article[iv]* published by Daniel Boucek from DCIS who was a member of the workgroup. This article lists the policy changes that TMA/DHA brought to the table as

---

[8] Some of these conclusions are based on conversations with Mr. Boucek, the author of the article.

14

well as the single change DCIS and the other outside agencies made. Those outside TMA/DHA were concerned that some measures brought to the table by TMA/DHA would result in access to care issues which, years later, have proven to be true and finally even TMA/DHA admitted to those failures but still offer no alternatives while avoiding the recommendation made by the outside groups.[9]

Due to administrative actions implemented by TMA/DHA, HVC ceased operation in 2005. The first administrative action was to secretly freeze all claims that involved about 95% of all major hospitals in the Philippines and their contractor was forbidden to tell beneficiaries that called asking why their claims were being held; this went on for many months before we were able to get it stopped. We were informed by TMA/DHA that this was done in order to try to collect money due the government for past fraud involving HVC. It was obvious TMA/DHA had little understanding of how HVC operated so assumed, wrongly, that hospitals that HVC contracted with to provide inpatient care were involved in the fraud. While that was true for a limited number of hospitals owned by HVC, they had no intention of sharing their profits with others. In reality they paid local hospitals cash or made credit arrangements at local prevailing rates. Then turned around and manufactured a bill in the name of the hospital but at HVC's address at rates many times higher than actually paid. I passed this information on to MG Granger when I became aware of the freeze. He said his staff assured him that only a few beneficiaries would be affected by the freeze but I was able to show him otherwise and explained how HVC really worked. Within days he had the freeze lifted and beneficiaries finally started to get reimbursed for legitimate care they had paid for. In 2007 they started to implement the various new restrictions brought forward in the workgroup on the now unique TRICARE Philippine Standard.

Workgroup Changes

- Supplemental insurance plans
- Legislative changes to sanction beneficiaries

---

[9] On page 15 of the DODIG report 2014-052, (http://www.dodig.mil/pubs/documents/DODIG-2014-052.pdf) The Assistant Secretary stated that while health care costs have decreased in Panama and the Philippines, TRICARE Standard beneficiaries have experienced a negative impact on access to care and increased out-of-pocket costs. Our own survey and analysis of cost data support these contentions as well and were relayed to TMA/DHA years ago.

- Third party billing
- Cap coverage and adequacy
- Increased use of medical reviews on claims
- Creation of a network

Each of these is discussed below with the exception of supplemental insurance plans. I am unaware of any actions taken in this direction other than a short discussion concerning TMA/DHA offering to fund a local plan selected by beneficiaries in lieu of using TRICARE Standard but that was years ago.

Legislative Changes to Sanction Beneficiaries

TMA/DHA requested authority to terminate beneficiaries TRICARE benefit for around 5 years if TMA/DHA felt they were involved in fraud. As far as we know there were no provisions for appeal. Fortunately Congress denied the request.

Third Party Billing

One of the processes used by HVC to defraud was to pay local physicians and hospitals for care provided to TRICARE beneficiaries and then file claims on their behalf at their address but for amounts well in excess of the local rates they paid. This is what TMA/DHA saw as "third party billing". In the U.S. third party billing is where a health care provider contracts with a company to complete the documents required for filing their claims for an agreed amount and the payer would send the money to the provider. In the Philippines what they saw as third party billing was the practice initiated by HVC and copied by others that was aided by ISOS for a fee after HVC was closed. Only one aspect of this practice was addressed. That being inpatient claims. The rule change required all hospital reimbursements to be sent to the address of record of the hospital. This pretty much stopped this aspect of the fraud but neglected the same fraud with respect to outpatient care. We did see evidence that ISOS tried to circumvent this policy at one hospital but it failed.

Cap Coverage and Adequacy

Historically TMA/DHA paid and continues pay billed charges overseas. Many Philippine providers, following the example from HVC, continued to charge rates much above local rates. A table of maximum allowable charges, Champus Maximum Allowed Charge

(CMAC), was developed in an attempt to limit payments to local rates. To do this TMA/DHA decided to use World Bank International Comparison Program (ICP) Purchasing Power Parity (PPP) rates to determine the percentage of TMA/DHA developed U.S. average charges for procedures. They called the PPPs "country specific index factors". To apply these rates, bills paid in Philippine pesos are converted to dollars using a reduced exchange rate on the date of care. Then the dollar amount is compared to the CMAC. If the converted dollar amount is higher than the CMAC, the amount over the rate is deducted and the result is called the "allowed amount".

Even before implementation they found, with our help, that the rate from the World Bank calculations was not going to work. It showed that no one at TMA/DHA tried to verify their conclusions. Many articles on the PPP rates suggested using detailed comparisons between a 3rd world country and a 1st world country was problematic and not recommended but TMA/DHA chose to ignore those cautions.

Because of our work it was found that a single percentage would not work across all segments of care so major adjustments were made. First the overall PPP rate was increased from 22.9% to 52%. Second ancillary rates were set at the Puerto Rico rates and high cost inpatient procedures were carved out and given higher per diem rates for the hospital charges. These two significant increases over their original concept in themselves proved the concept was flawed. Instead of rates tailored to regions like in the U.S. one rate was used for the entire Philippines which also showed that nobody at TMA/DHA did any real research into local medical rates. The result was one size fits all from urban to rural.

Increased Use of Medical Reviews on Claims

This program is called "Prepayment Review" and the stated purpose is to review medical necessity or appropriate level of care or amounts billed. This is what TMA/DHA has to say about prepayment review.

"The review process may require the provider [or beneficiary] to submit additional information such as medical documentation associated with the claim. Prepayment review is one of the most effective anti-fraud controls available. This control helps ensure

appropriate expenditure of government dollars, avoiding the 'pay and chase problem' of getting dollars back after they are paid."

Creation of a Network

The original intent of this change as envisioned by the proponents of the change and as addressed in the *article*[v] by Daniel Boucek of DCIS was a contract with a local national HMO/PPO. Instead TMA/DHA decided to create their own which started in 2013. It was created by their contractor ISOS and limits care to a very few providers who are chosen based only on their agreement to participate; no quality checks are accomplished. The contractor was responsible to train providers and all beneficiaries across the Philippines about this unique but limited program that applies in less than 2% of the Philippines and even in these areas only part time. It was phased in across this 2% over an 18 month period in what was called Phase I, II and III. Essentially any beneficiary that receives care within the geographic boundaries of this 2% of the Philippines is required to follow the rules of what they call the Philippine Demonstration Project, Demo for short.

The Consequences Resulting from the TMA/DHA Modifications to the Philippine Benefit

The lack of firsthand knowledge of the Philippine culture and health care industry practices, processes and culture was and continues to be a major roadblock to TMA/DHA's ability to manage the medical benefit in the Philippines. Not knowing where the beneficiary population lives also contributes to this problem.[10] MG Granger saw this problem and promised to place a TMA/DHA employee on the ground.

In 2008 the beneficiaries were promised an onsite employee that would listen to their issues and learn the nuances of the local health care industry so access to care could be restored.[11] Three years later in 2011 the *DODIG*[vi], as the result of a multi-year investigation of the contractor, recommended to TMA/DHA.

"Consider establishing a TRICARE presence in the Philippines to service military retirees and their dependents."

Their response was.

"TMA is in the process of selecting a location for a TRICARE Satellite Office in Manila, Philippines to provide assistance to military retirees and their dependents residing there. The office will be staffed by a TMA Government employee, and TMA is currently in the process of advertising that position."

Yet in 2013 there was still no such position and TMA/DHA continued to ignore beneficiary requests for information on the status.

In January 2014 the Director of DHA, Lt. Gen Robb, was to appear before a subcommittee of the House Armed Services Committee. My Congressman decided to present a written question asking, among other things, about the status of the long missing employee. The letter was submitted to the Director. His *response*[vii]

---

[10] See Philippine TRICARE Beneficiary Population Distribution Discussion (https://db.tt/1hxZOTUu) for a detailed explanation of the issue.

[11] Reference study (https://db.tt/ZgbPOill) that shows Philippine beneficiaries pay for most of their own care since DHA only expends about 13% of what they spend on all other beneficiaries.

contained statements that were not true, begged the question or that were misleading and intended to deceive Congress and beneficiaries. These covered various issues that will be addressed as the issues are addressed later. For now we will address those statements he made relevant to the missing government employee.

Two paragraphs deal with the promised government employee.

"In 2008, the Deputy Director, TRICARE Management Activity (TMA), visited the Republic of the Philippines. Based on what he saw and heard from the retired beneficiaries, as well as his awareness of significant fraud issues in the Philippines, the Deputy Director directed establishment of a satellite office in the Philippines to enable the TRICARE Area Office- Pacific to better support beneficiaries living there. At that time, office space was identified at the old Clark Air Force Base, and coordination was completed to have a U.S. citizen who would staff the office fall under the protection of the U.S. Embassy. Since that time, the space at the old Clark Air Force Base is no longer available."

and

"In 2012, the Deputy Director, TMA reversed the previous decision to establish a satellite office in the Philippines in light of several factors. These factors included the award of the TRICARE Overseas Program (TOP) contract in 2009 to International SOS Assistance (International SOS). This contract requires the operation of a 24/7 Regional Call Center, staffed with customer service representatives trained to assist beneficiaries and host nation providers with questions about claims, locating a provider, benefit determinations, and authorizations for care. Additionally, the agency had decided to implement the Philippine Demonstration Project which is designed to increase access to quality health care, eliminate the need for beneficiaries to file their own claims, and control costs. The Demonstration Project began in January 2013. Nowhere else do we have a TRICARE office specifically to support the retiree population in any other overseas location and establishing one in the Philippines would be potentially precedent-setting, resulting in

retirees living in other overseas locations expecting to have a satellite office established specifically to support them. And finally, in this resource constrained environment, establishing a satellite office in the Philippines was not a fiscally sound decision."

These two paragraphs are fraught with wrong, misleading or manufactured information.

1. The Deputy Director of TMA in 2008 was MG Elder Granger a longtime friend and who I spent many hours discussing the TRICARE issues in the Philippines; he retired in July 2009. He never visited the Philippines contrary to Lt. Gen Robb's claim above. Not only didn't he ever visit, his request to visit the Philippines in 2009 was denied. The truth is he decided to place an employee in the Philippines after my and other retiree recommendations and to accomplish two goals. The first was to have someone on the ground to monitor the effects of various policies/restrictions imposed by TMA/DHA and provide feedback so adjustments could be made to minimize loss of access to care. Second was to assisting beneficiaries with the complex requirements, unique to Philippine TRICARE, in converting claims from local global bills to U.S. itemized and costed bills.

2. The lost space at Clark was rented by TMA/DHA and remained vacant for years while TMA/DHA and the Embassy argued over the location. The Embassy refused to allow them to hire someone and place them at Clark due to security concerns. Finally TMA/DHA agreed to move the position to Manila and space was negotiated at the newly built VA clinic. This was three years later, in 2011, and at the same time, as they told the DODIG, they advertised the position for a second time.

3. The TOP contract and so called 24/7 Regional Call Center were a known quantity in 2008 when MG Granger agreed to the position and was not designed to duplicate but to compliment it with additional functions. In addition the

DODIG addressed this as well in 2011 well after the TOP contract start, implying it was insufficient when they said. *"Due to the absence of TMA resources in the Philippines, TRICARE beneficiaries must rely on phone calls and internet searches for information. Establishing a small TMA presence in the Philippines would provide an opportunity for TMA to educate both providers and beneficiaries. Beneficiaries would have a better outlet for resolving medical claim discrepancies and a direct means for reporting suspected fraudulent claims."*

So the claim that this newly discovered information removed the need for the position is felonious. In addition the DODIG made it clear that this was in addition to currently available resources and TMA/DHA responded that they concurred with the reasoning of the DODIG. Obviously TMA/DHA was well aware of the 2009 TOP contract and associated support as was the DODIG in 2011 when the *DODIG*[viii] called for the addition of this position. In addition the DODIG report specifically addressed significant issues with local providers understanding TRICARE policies and well after the TOP contract went into place. So while he said.

"This contract requires the operation of a 24/7 Regional Call Center, staffed with customer service representatives trained to assist beneficiaries and host nation providers with questions about claims, locating a provider, benefit determinations, and authorizations for care."

He knew full well that the contractor was not meeting those needs that the DODIG was addressing and to which TMA/DHA agreed. This claim is inconsistent with the facts and clearly is begging the question.

4. He also made this claim.

"Additionally, the agency had decided to implement the Philippine Demonstration Project which is designed to

increase access to quality health care, eliminate the need for beneficiaries to file their own claims, and control costs." This is nothing more than a false premise as the Demonstration was on the table and defined well before 2011. In fact included in the DODIG report is an acknowledgement that TMA/DHA was in the process of implementing the Demonstration and even listed the processes that were to be included. So both TMA/DHA and the DODIG knew of this project and considered it when the recommendation and concurrence were made. In addition the statement about increasing access to quality health care is totally felonious as the TOP contract does not require quality checks of providers and senior ISOS staff confirmed the only quality check was to use certified providers who they also admitted were not checked for quality. Further the claim that the Demonstration would eliminate the need for beneficiaries to file their own claims is also a false premise since at least 40% of the beneficiaries in the Philippines reside outside the 2% of the Philippines that is covered by the Demonstration. In addition the majority of specialties within the Demonstration areas carry waivers that require beneficiaries in these areas to revert to the alternate and limited Philippine TRICARE Overseas Standard. This is also the case whenever the 60% that are in the Demonstration areas travel. The reality is thousands of claims are still filed by beneficiaries unless, like many, they opt to pay for their own care because they feel that their claims will not be paid anyway.[12]

Certification of Providers

This process was implemented well before the HVC fraud came on the scene and as addressed earlier indirectly lead to increased fraud

---

[12] Our survey (https://db.tt/ExzpuQfR) of military retirees living in the Philippines clearly showed that a significant number no longer file claims because of their past experiences where the claims were denied on a technicality or because they were not able to itemize and code their claims.

by pushing beneficiaries to find alternatives to paying for their care and submitting claims.

Although I was able to get TMA/DHA to produce an actual list of certified providers, the quality of the information was extremely poor. The specialty field was usually left blank, addresses were of little or no value. In many cases the address would be a street name or the name of a building or even just a barangay name. Often the province field was blank as was on occasion the city field.[13] Other times the listed city was wrong. There were no rules on data input so a city name may appear as "Angeles", "Angeles City", or even "Angeles Pampanga". In one instance one city had 7 different names in the database. There were no phone numbers which meant that one had to travel to each provider on the list, try to find the clinic based on an obscure address and then determine the provider's specialty. If it turned out to be the specialty they were looking for then, hopefully, they could determine what days and hours the clinic operated by looking at a sign on the door. If the provider was the wrong specialty they went to the next one on the list. Many times the same provider was listed at the same location but with different versions of his name.

In addition provider names were often misspelled or inverted. Sometimes the provider name is listed as "First, Middle, Last". Other times as, "Last, First, Middle" or "Last, Middle, First". Most of the time but not always no spaces were used. For example a Dr. Ralph Walter Randall would appear as "Randall,Ralph,Walter,M.D." or as "Randall,Walter,Ralph,M.D." or even "Randall,Ralph Walter,M.D." Knowing if the name was correct or what the real name was became a major task.

After about seven years of requesting the database be cleaned up and being told to be patient we were finally able to get some incremental improvements in the data in 2012. Specialties were added as well as phone numbers and cities were standardized over a period of about six months. But names continue to this day without the

---

[13] Many cities and towns in the Philippines go by the same name. Without a province listed beneficiaries had little idea on which island the provider was located.

proper use of spaces or commas and duplicate entries are still common.

As mentioned earlier when TMA/DHA started to apply their new and Philippine unique rules they attempted to change some of the certification rules to preclude some of the processes used by HVC and their replacements that came on the scene with the help of ISOS, in many cases.

The first rule change was to alter the policy on payment of inpatient claims by sending payments to the address of record for the hospital instead of the address noted on the claim which was usually one of the questionable "physician groups". During this time I was involved with multiple providers through my Rotary and also knew of the existence of some of the "physician groups" in the area. I was also interested in who was certified in my area so I could use them when needed. So I checked the certified list each time it came out which varied from 30 to 60 days between updates. I noticed that the local private hospital, which had previously been certified, was dropped from the list. I called ISOS in Manila and was passed to the Director for the TRICARE operation. I asked why Mother Seton Hospital was no longer on the certified list. He asked me to wait while he checked the file and after a few minutes came back and said I would have to talk to this employee who managed my area. He said he was not in the office that day and suggested I call back the next day. I did and the individual told me that Mother Seton Hospital had violated the rules of certification by giving their certification number to a defrauder who was filing false claims.[14] He went on to assure me that he was coming to Naga in a few weeks and was going to talk to management at the hospital about this violation of policy and then reissue a new certification. I waited for a couple of months and rechecked the certified list only to find they were still not certified.

I decided to talk to the hospital administrator myself this time. I was directed to see the manager of the business office, a nun who agreed to see me. She explained that the hospital had decided not to be involved with TRICARE because they saw it as a corrupt and

---

[14] The defrauder he was referring to was a physician group owned by a businessman who ISOS had certified. While he claimed the problem was the hospital, no action was taken against this group who was submitting the false claims and they continued without interference from ISOS for years. Why will become clear as you read the book.

fraudulent program and wanted nothing to do with that. She went on to point out that when HVC was the "official representative" of TRICARE they had run up huge bills in local hospitals and then failed to pay. As mentioned earlier TMA/DHA stopped paying claims for HVC which caused them to close. Because HVC was seen as the official representative of TRICARE these hospitals blamed TRICARE and the U.S. government for their losses.[15] Because of that they no longer granted credit to TRICARE patients. She said that a number of TRICARE patients used a local group known as the Retired US Military Service Healthcare Philippines Inc. This group was certified by ISOS and brought patients to them for hospitalization and paid cash when the patient was discharged. She said this group advised her that due to a change by TRICARE, the claims they submitted to be reimbursed for the cost of the inpatient care would be sent to the hospital and told them whenever they received a letter from the TRICARE claims contractor to call them and they would pick it up. After doing this for a short time they became suspicious and opened one of the letters. They were surprised to find an EOB and check for an amount well above the actual cost of the care. So they made a copy of the actual hospital bill and sent it all back to Wisconsin Physicians Service (WPS) explaining the amount paid was well over the actual amount and that they did not bill TRICARE so to please stop sending these checks to them. They did this a number of times but the checks just kept coming so they asked ISOS to remove them from the certified list. They told me that ISOS did come to talk to them about recertification but said it was a requirement that they agree to file claims or allow others to file claims for them as part of certification and refused. This story was significantly different from what ISOS told me and they refused to consider certification.[16]

---

[15] I addressed this issue with TMA/DHA about how many Philippine providers saw HVC and TRICARE as one and the same and there was a need to set the record straight. They didn't seem interested so this misconception continues to this day to the detriment of beneficiaries.

[16] About a year later I was able to convince them that things were different and I would assist them in reporting any further acts of fraud. I was able to get MG Granger to agree to call and talk to them if necessary but they agreed to certification if I was present. The TAO-P contacted ISOS and directed them to send the director to do the certification and I met him at the hospital. By this time the fraud involving them had been exposed, addressed later, and he knew I was involved. He was very curious as to what specifically I knew about the fraud. I told him he was there and should know more than me but he said he was interested in what I knew to see if I knew something he didn't. I refused to discuss it with him.

I started to investigate these groups because I wanted to understand how they were able to bypass the processes that were supposed to preclude their existence as TRICARE providers. I visited the group mentioned above and they wanted me to use them for care. I told them I would not agree to sign blank claim forms nor would I sign claims where the amount billed was substantially higher than the local rates paid. They said they didn't do that so I agreed. For a year I received care from physicians and medications and was never asked to sign a claim form of any sort and never received any EOBs for this timeframe.

Around this same time another policy change was implemented that TMA/DHA claimed was to further limit third party billing. That policy required certified providers be certified at every clinic physical location. Unlike in the states where most physicians operate from one and sometimes two clinic locations, local physicians offer clinics in multiple locations and it is not uncommon to see a physician with 4 or 5 locations where they offer a few hours of clinic a week. This had the potential of doubling or tripling the workload and cost for TMA/DHA for certification and I'm sure did. It is my understanding this recommendation came from ISOS as well. It would also be a major factor in how these questionable but certified physician groups could succeed in billing for care they had not provided and at rates 2 to 4 times above customary rates.

Sometime later the owner of the group approached me asking if I was interested in becoming a partner in the business as he said he needed additional funds. I told him I needed to know how the business worked before I could consider it. I saw this as an opportunity to find out how these groups could exist and be paid but had no intention of becoming involved. I was walked through the entire process including how ISOS certified them as a "physician group" without any physicians present.

"Physician group" is a classification of provider on the certified list; this would become clearer when I obtained seven years of the actual ISOS database. ISOS used this classification to inappropriately certify businessmen and single physicians as large physician groups. As explained to me a businessman could apply to ISOS to be certified as a physician group. Once that certification took place the group would use local physicians to see their patients by taking them to their local offices and paying for the visit. They asked the physician to do a second SOAP entry on the group's letterhead explaining that the patient was part of an HMO and they needed it for their records.[17] They would then contact ISOS who would certify the provider using the physician group's address and without visiting the provider.[18] This allowed the group to file a claim for the physician visit but in their name and for amounts well above local rates.

Interaction with my forum members showed these physician groups were springing up all over the Philippines and obviously with the cooperation of ISOS and they functioned in the same manner as the old HVC but on a local and smaller scale. This allowed them to pay for care at hospitals and local physicians and be reimbursed at much higher rates to their address. The new rule requiring multiple certifications of a provider by clinic location helped to facilitate this process and its implementation seemed more than a coincidence. But their ability to be reimbursed for inpatient care had been curtailed so most of them no longer provided for inpatient care.

I tried to address to TMA/DHA the new change to certification that required providers be certified at each location and tried to point out how that was being used to the advantage of defrauders. I was still not fully aware of just how involved ISOS was in this process but knew the new policy made it easier, not harder, to file false claims. I was essentially told ISOS knew more than I about the fraud so no action was taken to correct this loophole.

Around this time the TMA/DHA implemented a charge master which limited the amounts paid for care. This charge master was called the CHAMPUS Maximum Allowable Charge or CMAC. Prior to this they paid billed charges in the Philippines as they did and continue to do for TRICARE Prime Remote in the Philippines as well as all TRICARE beneficiaries in other countries.[19] This will be discussed in more detail later but this process started to limit the amounts these physician groups could claim and how to file claims.

It wasn't too long after that the owner of the group that wanted me to become a partner called me and asked me to meet him and he

---

[17] SOAP is an acronym for Subjective, Objective, Assessment, and Plan and a method of documenting patient encounters by physicians.

[18] Since these providers did not see patients at the certified provider group address, ISOS was unable to do a physical encounter at the address listed for the provider.

[19] A CMAC was later implemented in Panama but with more liberal payment rates. In spite of that they also have major access to care issues which are also the result of this change.

28

seemed quite upset. When I met him he told me in detail how he was certified. Apparently ISOS was willing to certify anyone that didn't meet the requirements for the right fee. In his case he paid a fee each time his certification came up for renewal. When the group was certified apparently the fee also included certifying any provider they wanted as being part of their group. Then the CMAC came into play and apparently ISOS saw an opportunity to make more money. The fee increased but included in the higher fee was training on how to file claims using the CMAC and a copy of the CMAC was provided along with a bootleg copy of the American Medical Association CPT manual; all on CD. Essentially they taught them how to file claims at the highest rate the CMAC would allow and because it was built using U.S. billing practices it overstated local visit fees by up to five fold.[20] What had the owner upset was he was notified by ISOS that the fee schedule was changing and he would no longer be charged fee at recertification but a fee based on a percentage of his reimbursements from TRICARE. He said that was unfair and asked me if I could intervene for him. I asked him the name of the ISOS employee he dealt with and he told me. To further confirm what he told me I visited a woman I knew that used to work for a similar group in the area and told her what I knew. She wasn't aware of the new fee increase but said the fees had been in place for a long time and further said she was aware this was going on in other locations in the Philippines as some of the groups tried to expand to new areas outside southern Luzon.

I reported what I knew to a TMA/DHA employee. He said he had heard they were selling bootleg coding manuals and thought they had stopped. After some time without hearing anything back I contacted him again and was told ISOS claimed it was an isolated incident involving a single employee who was fired. I tried to point out that I was told this was Philippine wide and given the number of apparent provider groups that were certified and using the same process across the Philippines it was unlikely to have been an isolated incident because ISOS used different employees in different regions. I was told TMA/DHA was satisfied with ISOS's explanation and I was not to speak of the incident again.

---

[20] While outpatient fees are grossly overstated, many ancillary services and surgical fees are grossly understated.

Another certification practice, which came to light through my forum, was physicians were being certified as hospitals so they could file fake hospital claims and be paid. Based on these reports I personally used one of them to watch the process and keep track of the actual costs involved in the care since the retiree that reported it on the group said he reported the fraudulent certifications and claims but no action was taken by TMA/DHA. These physicians advertised around St. Luke's that they were TRICARE's representative and if a beneficiary agreed to use their services and sign a blank claim form they would cover the costs of inpatient care at St. Luke's and file a claim. In my case they paid the costs of my care and then filed a claim for about ten times more than the actual cost of the care including claiming care that was never received. The day the EOB was posted on the WPS web page and days before a check was cut and mailed I contacted them and advised them that they should not send the check as the claim was inflated and contained claims for care never received. I was ignored and the check sent. Only after months of extensive follow-up and threats of going public did TMA/DHA finally remove this single provider from the certified list. But they ignored the many other physicians that openly advertised the same service around St. Luke's and they were allowed to file fraudulent claims for years even though I pointed out to TMA/DHA that my example was only one of many. I also pointed out to TMA/DHA that something must be seriously wrong with their claims payment process that allowed a single physician's office to file claims as a tertiary hospital with all the attached services and suggested someone needed to look into how this could happen.

Only later, when I obtained seven years of the actual ISOS certified provider database, was it clear that these physicians were able to do this because ISOS had certified them as hospitals and not physicians and it was also clear that TMA/DHA ignored my recommendation to look into how physicians could bill and be paid as a hospital. Again I addressed the issue of physicians billing and being paid as a hospital to TMA/DHA along with this new evidence. Once again I was ignored and the practice continued unabated.

During a conversation with a senior investigator from DCIS who said he was aware of this practice but was unable to figure out how it was done asked me if I knew how they did it. I explained the process including how ISOS was involved by certifying them as a hospital instead of a physician and how unlikely it was that it was a mistake since they were required to obtain and file a copy of their license which did not exist in these cases. I explained how they could identify those involved. I also told him about the practice of certifying single physicians and businessmen as provider groups. He told me he could not discuss this in the future if an investigation resulted.

Not long after that I noticed the physician hospitals quietly disappeared from the list and one by one the physician groups also disappeared. Although I had moved a few years earlier one of the groups where I knew some of the staff contacted me because they found they had been summarily removed from the certified list and asked if I could help them understand what happened. I suggested they contact ISOS and they received a response that they were removed because they were wrongly certified as "institutional" and if they wanted to be certified again they needed to file a claim. That was done but they were still denied certification. Of note all the providers in the area that ISOS had previously certified at the groups address were also removed for that address but their real addresses remained.

Not long after that *DODIG Report No. D-2011-107*[ix], Improvements Needed in Procedures for Certifying Medical Providers and Processing and Paying Medical Claims in the Philippines came out and made everything clear to me. The reports objective stated;

"We conducted this audit as a result of internal control deficiencies identified while supporting the Defense Criminal Investigative Service (DCIS) and the U.S. Attorney's Office, Western District of Wisconsin. The objectives were to evaluate management controls over procedures for certifying medical providers treating military retirees and their dependents in the Philippines and to review selected procedures for processing and paying Philippine medical claims."

The timing of the DCIS investigation addressed in this report to my conversation with the DCIS investigator and the quiet removal of the providers made it clear to me what happened and what the real findings were. As usual with DCIS findings they were never made public and any penalties if any imposed on the offending contractor. What I had reported to TMA/DHA for years but ignored finally resulted in the removal of these certified providers. And given the information presented above it should be clear to you as well.

Between the TMA/DHA polices that reduced access to care and payment of claims and the contractor facilitating questionable certifications, fraud just kept marching on. When these fraudulent providers were reported little happened. TMA/DHA, at one point, even recommended these groups as places to go to receive care where they would submit claims for beneficiaries.[21]

While the certified provider list eventually became a little more usable it was still one of the primary TMA/DHA policies that drove beneficiaries to use defrauders; better to pay a little higher co-pay than to pay the full amount. We know from experience that ISOS takes as long as seven months to certify a provider; the contract specifies 60 days. I have personal experience where ISOS claimed legitimate providers didn't exist, denying the certification. If a provider did not exist than the claim must be fraudulently filed but TMA/DHA have never file charges. In one instance when they claimed two providers did not exist and two claims were denied it turned out they failed to go to the addresses noted on the claim nor did they take any action to confirm the existence of the providers and denied the claims.

We could not use local chain pharmacies because TMA/DHA only allowed single locations to be certified which meant a beneficiary may have to drive by two or three of the same pharmacies to get to the one certified in the area. Only recently and after years of suggesting providers such as pharmacies be certified at the corporate level did TMA/DHA finally relent. But they stopped after only a couple chains were certified and after they found that two major chains refused to deal with them. That resulted in the total loss of all outlets of both chains; Manson Drug and South Star Pharmacy. In

---

[21] These groups continued to operate for many years and thought they are legitimate because TMA/DHA failed to follow up and reeducate them and they saw ISOS as the TRICARE authority. In fact I was told just that by one group when I suggested they were committing fraud. They responded by saying, "If what we do is fraud why did TRICARE's company here show us how to do it? Who are you to tell us we are committing fraud". They were easy to find by searching groups and identifying those that routinely bill at the maximum allowed amount or more. From my experience legitimate groups bill at local rates, at least the ones that didn't learn the practice from ISOS. During the implementation of the CMAC many of us were concerned many of the rates were to low and would not cover the local costs. TMA/DHA advised us to use providers that filed claims so we wouldn't bear the cost of disallowed amounts. We asked them to provide a list of these providers and they gave us a list that contained most of the known defrauders certified by ISOS. So in practice TMA/DHA recommended we use defrauders that their contractor legitimized even after we reported them as such.

addition the problems with providers that previously declined certification, who are not contacted again, continues to cause claims to be denied as do all the other idiosyncrasies involved with a secret policy like this. This is not true for active duty and their dependents that live in the Philippines as they have a comprehensive list comparable to those in the U.S. which speaks volumes to how TMA/DHA sees retirees as second class citizens.[22]

It is interesting to see how Lt. Gen Robb begs the questions on certification in his *response*[x] to the House Armed Services Committee with regard to the issue of national certification of pharmacies, the Philippine Red Cross and major hospitals in the southern Philippines.

In his first paragraph he says;

"All three of the major national pharmacy firms operating in the Republic of the Philippines are TRICARE certified. Mercury Drug was certified in September 2010; Rose Pharmacy in April 2012; and

---

[22] A review of seven years of the Certified Provider database shows an average of about 100 legitimate providers a year were not certified due to declination by the provider and not because they were not licensed providers. Since certification doesn't start until a claim is filed that represents at least 100 claims a year that were denied. During this same seven year period a total of only 59 certifications were denied due the entity not being a legitimate provider and it appears, based on the names of the businesses, that claims were filed for medical equipment purchased from them such as a hardware store. We were later able to get these kinds of businesses certified but many legitimate claims were denied in the interim. In reality significantly fewer than 59 were denied certification for truly legitimate reasons. During the same period 712 were denied because they refused to be certified. The process is kept secret from beneficiaries so they are not able to assist in persuading providers to agree to certification. Whenever we ask to be provided with the specific process and requirements of certification or the causes of non-certification of specific providers, ISOS claims the process is secret on the basis it is really a medical quality assurance review. But we know that only basic clerks with a check list, as outlined in the referenced DODIG report above, are used for certification. Further we know that the TRICARE Operations Manual states that the TOP contractor is not required to do quality checks on providers overseas. Certification can cost a provider money so providers that see one TRICARE patient or so a month and don't associate them with the process see no reason to agree to certification. Beneficiaries are not allowed to know the outcome of the certification process. So if the provider was not certified because of previous declination, ISOS does not ask a second time but this is kept secret from the beneficiary. Also the policy in affect for years of denying claims that were submitted where the provider is not already certified and not informing the beneficiary that once the provider was certified they could resubmit the claim was a major issue. A conservative estimate of two thousand additional instances of care was paid for by the beneficiary each year due to this failure by TMA/DHA. It doesn't take to many denials before people look to someone that will provide their care as was promised. Later we were able to get TMA/DHA to modify the process so that claims were held 90 days pending certification of the provider and we used our assets to publicize the new policy and how a claim could be resubmitted once a provider was certified as TMA/DHA didn't feel it was necessary to publicize that information.

Watsons Pharmacy in July 2013. *Certification of these pharmaceutical companies at the corporate level allow TRICARE beneficiaries to access any of these pharmacies' stores, regardless of where in the country they are located. The Philippine National Red Cross is TRICARE certified effective February 19, 2014. Similar to the certification of the pharmacy companies, certification of the Red Cross at the national level allows TRICARE beneficiaries to access any of the 80 Red Cross Chapters in the Philippines to obtain the necessary testing and blood supplies they may need. Due to the delay in certifying the Philippine National Red Cross, the Defense Health Agency has directed the TRICARE Overseas Program contractor to reprocess all previously submitted claims since September 2010 and provide the appropriate reimbursement to the beneficiaries for their out of pocket expenses for testing and blood supplies obtained from any Philippine Red Cross chapter."*

This is followed with one sentence buried at the end of the last paragraph that states;

"Additionally, throughout the Philippines there are 301 certified institutional facilities that provide inpatient services and 4,335 individual certified providers."

The original questions were: *"Major national pharmacy firms and the Red Cross and all of its field offices have refused to work with the contractor denying beneficiary access to numerous pharmacies and a major source of blood. One of four internationally accredited hospitals and the only one in the southern Philippines cannot be used by beneficiaries for what appears to be nothing more than a paperwork exercise as it is obviously a licensed and legitimate hospital with better quality than many currently certified hospitals."*

1. Declaring that all three of the major national pharmacy firms are certified simply begged the question which dealt with why major national pharmacy firms refused to work with the contractor. Two major national pharmacy firms, Manson Drug and South Star Pharmacy have refused to work with ISOS and are no longer available to beneficiaries. That was the issue he should have addressed. He didn't even get the dates of national certification right but real facts don't seem to be of concern to TMA/DHA; Mercury Drug was not nationally certified in 2010. It wasn't until mid-2011 when I brought up

the subject yet again while at Tripler in Hawaii that a TMA/DHA employee agree to talk to ISOS again to see if they would agree; we pushed this approach for 5 years before it happened. In the past ISOS turned down the idea as not feasible. But then they were paid by certification plus travel costs where, now the contract had been changed and they were paid a fixed annual fee. My belief is this was the real incentive that finally allowed this process to go forward.

In addition, at the time the question was posed to the director, the Red Cross and all of its field offices had refused to cooperate with ISOS on certification. I was advised we would have to find alternative sources of blood as it would not be certified. External publicity apparently forced TMA/DHA to direct ISOS to certify the Red Cross based on its international certification rather than a local check of the provider since within days of this exposure the denied certification of the Red Cross and all its chapters was reversed. When you consider normal certifications take 90 days or more for a single location, this was a significant event. For as long as certification was required claims from the Red Cross have been denied. Only when I raised the issue of these denied claims and certification with a now deceased WWII Filipino-American retiree and was told of the refusal to cooperate was the issue made public through our blog. Per my recommendation in the blog one or more retirees contacted the Armed Services Blood Program on Facebook asking if they might provide blood to TRICARE beneficiaries in the Philippines because of the certification denial. I know that they brought this to the attention of TMA/DHA and within days the denial was reversed and probably set a record for certification, let alone a national certification with hundreds of chapters spread throughout the country. The comment about the delay in certification prompted a directive to reprocess all previously denied claims shows two things. One, if it is to be believed, ISOS was negligent in certifying the Red Cross for 4 years. Since the relook was really the result of my raising this issue and the denied WWII retirees' 2010 claim and suggesting that they relook these claims it seems TMA/DHA is trying to mislead the public in the real truth behind this recent certification reversal and retroactive payments.

2. The second certification issue posed in the question referenced the failure to certify an internationally accredited hospital while certifying others with much lower quality. This question was ignored completely. Instead of answering the question the General bypassed the question by listing statics that were not relevant to the original question. So the question remains unanswered. This was nothing more than begging the question instead of providing a real response to the issue at hand. We know, based on responses from ISOS and TMA/DHA and reviewing the TRICARE Operations Manual (TOM) that quality of providers is not a concern when selecting overseas providers and many of the hospitals that are certified lack facilities that westerners have come to expect. But they may be the only hospital in an area. See this video *example*[xi] of the kind of hospitals that TMA/DHA accepts for their Demonstration. The real issue still exists and high quality internationally accredited hospitals still remain uncertified due to a *paperwork exercise gone bad.*[xii]

Cap Coverage and Adequacy

Historically TMA/DHA paid billed charges overseas and still does everywhere but in the Philippines and Panama. TMA/DHA complained for many years that local providers were adding additional fees or increasing their fees above what local patients paid when billing TRICARE patients. So a charge master known as the Champus Maximum Allowed Charge (CMAC) was developed in an attempt to limit payments to local rates. To do this TMA/DHA decided to use World Bank International Comparison Program (ICP) Purchasing Power Parity (PPP) rates to determine the percentage of TMA/DHA developed U.S. average charges for procedures. They called the PPPs "country specific index factors". To apply these rates, bills paid in Philippine pesos are converted to dollars using a reduced exchange rate on the date of care. Then the dollar amount is compared to the CMAC. If the converted dollar amount is higher than the CMAC, the amount over the rate is deducted and the result is called the "allowed amount". Based on the ICP PPPs and TMA/DHA's analyst's calculations the overall rate used to convert the average U.S. CMAC rates was 22.9%.

Simply put, it's based on an average local cost, Purchasing Power Parities (PPP), which was then converted to a percentage of what is spent in the U.S. for the same general services. The problem with the local average cost of medical care, however, is 45% of the population survive on less than a dollar a day and obtains their care in government hospitals where they pay almost nothing for their bed which is on a large ward. Families provide meals, linen, fans, IV kits or anything else ordered by the doctor as well as performing some nursing responsibilities and housekeeping chores which are not included in the cost. Physicians, seeing these patients, charge only a small fraction of what they charge patients in private hospitals. TRICARE beneficiaries use private hospitals that come closer to meeting U.S. standards, don't stay in large open wards and therefore pay higher rates for their hospital room and physician fees. So when averages, which include the cost of what the west would consider substandard care for a substantial portion of the local population, are used to calculate the maximum allowable charge it will not reflect the true cost of care for TRICARE beneficiaries which results in many instances of disallowed amounts for inpatient physician fees in particular but also in many other areas as well. If I, with the help of my group, had not been able to cause the substantial increase in the original PPP percentage from 22.9% to 52% of U.S. costs the disallowed amounts would be exponentially greater. Another significant error on the part of TMA/DHA was to apply the PPP for medical care, which is an average cost for a basket of goods and assume that the same percentage applies equally to more than 20,000 individual procedures. In addition to our ability to show, before the CMAC was ever implemented that the basic rate was seriously flawed, we demonstrated that ancillary rates were even more out of line with the 22.9%. In fact so much so that they were set at 100% of the Puerto Rico rates. High cost inpatient procedures were carved out and given higher per diem rates for the hospital charges also because we demonstrated that their calculations were flawed. Instead of rates tailored to regions like in the U.S. where more than 90 CMACs are used, one rate was used for the entire Philippines which creates more problems.

This approach resulted in the following issues.

Requires beneficiaries to absorb the cost of lower exchange rates

Instead of developing the CMAC in local currency it was developed in dollars. This requires the claims processor to first convert the local cost in pesos to dollars using the current exchange rate, minus about 2%[23], before comparing to the CMAC. When the CMAC was first designed beneficiaries received more than 50 pesos to the dollar and comparisons with actual charges during that time were used in part to set the 52% percentage. In 2013 beneficiaries received about 42.4 pesos to the dollar. This means beneficiaries are required to absorb the higher cost of the peso.

If the valuation between the two currencies were reversed the net affect would have been to increase the effective CMAC rates which could be exploited by third party billers, increasing fraud. Beneficiaries in other overseas areas are not required to absorb the cost of a lower exchange rate. This policy does nothing to reduce fraud and may increase fraud by driving beneficiaries to use billers and others that bill TRICARE but find ways to overcharge.

CMAC is not adjusted for Philippine inflation

U.S. inflation is used as the basis for changing CMAC rates instead of Philippine inflation. Each year the updated Philippine CMAC is based on the percentages addressed earlier and applied to the new U.S. average CMAC. According to the *World Bank*[xiii], inflation in the Philippines from 2008 through 2013 was 18.8% while in the U.S. it was 8% or an increase of 10.8% over U.S. inflation.

Consequences Due to the TMA/DHA Approach

When the CMAC was being developed the exchange rate was more than 50 pesos to the dollar. In 2013 it was 42.4 pesos to the dollar or 15.2% lower. Between inflation and the exchange rate, the dollar value of the CMAC dropped by 26%. I addressed this issue for

---

[23] By contract WPS uses exchange rates from Citibank at about 2% below the actual rate. This translates into higher dollar conversions which means larger amounts are unfairly classified as above the maximum allowed amount.

years with TMA/DHA and was advised that they did annual evaluations of these differences and made any necessary adjustments. When I asked to see copies of these evaluations in 2013 I was told they were classified. However a few months later and apparently after reviewing the information I sent they increased the 52% rate to 54% which only represented a 2% adjustment to the 26% reduction in value and caused absolutely no increase for pharmacy and ancillary procedures which were already at 100%. Another issue not considered by TMA/DHA is cost deflation of some procedures in the U.S. that are not reflected in the Philippines where prices are not driven by Medicare and other U.S. policies.

These increases in cost have most acutely been felt in the ancillary, outpatient surgical and inpatient professional fee areas. Beneficiaries in other overseas areas are not required to absorb the cost of inflation or exchange rate changes. This policy does nothing to reduce fraud in the Philippines.

						2008			2013	
							Actual			Actual	
			Convert	Convert to	CMAC	Patient Cost		CMAC	Patient Cost	
			to $ 2008	$ 2012	Allowed	Copay +		Allowed	Copay +	
		Local	50/1	42.4/1	Amount	disallowed	% Patient	Amount	disallowed	% Patient
CPT	Procedure	Charge	minus 2%	minus 2%	2008	amount	Paid	2013	amount	Paid
74150	CT KUB	PHP 10,560	$215.51	$254.14	$214.23	$54.84	25.45%	$133.90	$153.71	60.48%
93000	ECG	PHP 600	$12.24	$14.44	$10.25	$4.56	37.22%	$10.47	$6.59	45.62%
85027	CBC	PHP 471	$9.61	$11.34	$9.41	$2.55	26.58%	$9.48	$4.23	37.28%

This table shows the effects on the CMAC rates for changes in the exchange rate only. The 2% exchange adjustment reduces the actual rate by 2%. The new rate is used to convert the peso charge to dollars. If the inflation increase of more than 10% was taken into consideration the amount and percentage paid by beneficiaries would be significantly higher. Of note is in these random examples the actual CMAC rate for one procedure went from $214 to $134 a reduction of 37% while the cost of CT procedures has continued to increase in the Philippines. One reason for higher ancillary costs in the Philippines is the additional cost to transport the equipment to the Philippines plus the higher cost of supplies and maintenance and the lower amortization rates due to lower utilization.

Even the ECG rate increase of 2% and 0.7% for a CBC didn't keep up with U.S. inflation which was 8%. In reality the U.S. CMAC rates are driven by Medicare and other political factors as much as by inflation so trying to use them as a basis to build a Philippine CMAC has never been viable.

Built for U.S. medical billing practices and relationships; does not address regional differences

The CMAC for the Philippines uses averages to create one national set of fees, unlike in the U.S. where there are hundreds of sets of fees based on geographic area, urban vs. rural, sole community hospital, training mission, local cost of living etc. What this means in practice is that some of the rates are lower than the real local rates in high costs areas such as Manila while they are higher than in lower cost areas such as the provinces

The practical result is increased cost for the taxpayer and the beneficiary. For example a beneficiary that finds amounts on his claim from a high cost area are partially disallowed due to the fees exceeding the CMAC will be required to pay his co-pay based on the allowed amount plus pay the entire disallowed amount making his effective cost much higher than it should be. On the other hand a local provider that bills TRICARE is free to charge at the CMAC in the province where the actual local rates maybe 30% lower, making a huge profit at the expense of the taxpayer. While ancillary and surgical procedure rates are significantly lower than local customary rates, outpatient encounter rates are significantly higher and allows for significant overpayments which are occurring in the Demo. If a CMAC is to be implemented properly it has to be done using sample rates on the ground across multiple regions to develop locally appropriate fee schedules and tailored after local billing practices. In other words one size does not fit all, which is currently used and results in additional cost to the beneficiary and the taxpayer.

The current CMAC does not consider local global billing practices in the Philippines. Local custom is to provide the patient with a global bill for all services rendered. This is the norm and global bills are paid by local insurance companies using local billing practices. In the U.S. providers identify and cost all procedures in accordance with U.S. custom and law and which was used as the basis for the local CMAC design. This means local bills do not mesh with the CMAC and someone has to convert them under current policy. Providers are not equipped to identify all procedures in accordance with U.S. policies because they do not have ready access to the policy or trained coders and billers and further do not see procedures grouped or ungrouped in the same manner as the U.S. system requires. Most beneficiaries are likewise not equipped to do this.

Examples

A local provider sees outpatients and bills for the outpatient visit at the same rate regardless of how long they spend with the patient, the complexity of the problem or if additional procedures are accomplished. In the states a provider will bill established patients using a set of five medical codes that identify patients with longer visit times and complexities and the amounts billed increase with the complexity. They will also bill for any separate procedures accomplished such as a prostate exam which is not generally done in the Philippines as it is seen as an integral part of the visit. The CMAC is designed for this U.S. standard, not the Philippine standard, so does not properly reflect actual normal customary *fees*[xiv] in many instances.

A local provider treats a patient on an inpatient basis. He sets his fee based on the general condition of the patient and expected tasks required and on the type of hospital and room rate the patient chooses. In other words if the patient is admitted for an appendectomy and chooses a government hospital and an open ward the rate is significantly less than if the patient chooses an accredited private hospital and an upgraded private room. A secondary factor is the location of care. In high cost areas the fees are higher and in the provinces they are lower. On discharge his bill only reflects, "Professional Services" and an amount. In the U.S. DRGs are used but TMA/DHA uses individual procedures as the basis to reimburse for inpatient professional fees. In other words each time the doctor sees the patient he is required by TMA/DHA to charge a separate fee. Each surgical procedure is identified and charged at specific rates. On discharge TMA/DHA expects local providers to provide a uniquely U.S. bill that reflects a list of multiple procedures the physician performed during the inpatient stay and to cost them and within the TMA/DHA unique CMAC. Providers are not equipped to identify all procedures in accordance with U.S. policies because they do not have ready access to the policy or trained coders and billers and, further, do not see procedures grouped or ungrouped in the same manner as the U.S. system requires. Most beneficiaries are likewise not equipped to do this. This is not a problem in other countries as the claims processor simply identifies one or two procedures and assigns the global fee to those procedures and since billed charges are paid the entire bill will be paid. When they do that in the Philippines they only pay the CMAC rates for the one or two procedures they identify and the ten or twenty procedures they missed don't get paid or more often they deny the entire billed amount on the basis that the beneficiary failed to comply with their request and submit an itemized and costed bill.

The CMAC does not consider local professional fee setting. In the states a much larger percentage of a physician's income is derived from outpatient care as they charge at much higher rates, e.g. $15 in the Philippines vs. $100 in the U.S. for a visit. Inpatient fees make up a larger percentage of the physicians income in the Philippines. For example a doctor may charge $15 for an outpatient visit in the Philippines but charge $600 for a three day hospital stay for an appendectomy. In the states they may charge something like $100 for a visit and $1,000 for the three day hospital stay. In this example the local cost of an outpatient visit is 15% of the cost in the U.S. while the inpatient professional fees are 60% of the cost in the U.S. Therefore a CMAC based on a global percentage will overstate outpatient professional fees and understate inpatient professional fees and in particular surgical fees for both inpatient and outpatient settings in the Philippines. Anesthesiology is paid in the US based on minutes of service. In the Philippines it is billed as a percentage of the surgical fee; anywhere from 30 to 50 percent depending on location and hospital. Local insurance "CMAC's" are designed to accommodate the local billing system but since the TMA/DHA Philippine CMAC is designed for the U.S. billing system and practices it does not consider local practices which result in patients having large amounts disallowed as exceeding the maximum allowable charge. This only happens in the Philippines due to the CMAC and because it uses a simplistic average percentage method of converting the U.S. CMAC for Philippine billing and assumes overseas health care industry practices are identical to the U.S.

The bottom line of implementing a U.S. designed CMAC based on procedure level fees is that the average beneficiary has to learn medical coding and understand medical terminology in order to document individual procedures and cost those procedures for the contractor if they hope to get anything back from inpatient professional fees and more complex outpatient care beyond a basic visit. Once a beneficiary identifies each procedure they then must break out a typical global bill charge by procedure. To do this effectively they must first apply the proper CPT-4 code in order to look up the CMAC rate for the procedure. Then they must apply a reasonable amount of the global bill to the procedure. Even after doing this it is not unusual to find that some of the global bill remains which means at least that amount will be disallowed for payment consideration.

While this process is not explicitly required, failure to comply almost guarantees that claims for anything beyond a basic office visit or prescription will have most, if not all, the billed amount disallowed forcing the beneficiary to pay for most of all of their care.[24]

TMA/DHA will claim that beneficiaries do not need to break out claims. They also claim that a beneficiary can contact the contractor for assistance. In a response to a *Senator[xv]*, this is part of what they had to say.

"TRICARE beneficiaries who submit a claim for reimbursement to the TRICARE Overseas Claims Processor are required to complete the claim form DD 2642, Patient's Request for Medical Payment, and attach the following information that is normally provided by the provider on his or her letterhead:

1. Doctor's or provider's name/address (the one that actually provided the care). If there is more than one provider on the bill, circle his/her name;

2. Date of each service;

3. Place of each service;

4. Description of each surgical or medical service or supply furnished;

5. Charge for each service; and

6. The diagnosis should be included on the bill.

In general, this is the same information routinely included on an itemized bill from a provider."

This clearly shows how little they understand the local health care industry practices and customs. It shows that, in spite of what Lt. Gen Robb claimed when they cancelled the promised local position,

---

[24] See Professional Fee Processing Example (https://db.tt/ArxfRjKd) for a more graphic explanation of the differences between claims processing in the Philippines and the rest of the world.

there is a need for the position so TMA/DHA can learn local health care industry standards.

This is what they told the Senator about assistance beneficiaries could receive when filing claims from their contractor ISOS.

"TRICARE beneficiaries and host nation providers requiring assistance with claims may contact the TRICARE Overseas Program Regional Call Center at +65-6339-2676; beneficiaries should press option 2 and host nation providers should press option 5."

Our past experience shows that when we call the number above, we cannot trust what ISOS tells us and more often than not they tell us they don't have any answers but will call back. Then they are never heard from again. This experience is common with other beneficiaries as well. So instead of calling I email them so I have proof that they don't respond or what I was told when they do respond.

Here is what I asked and their response when I inquired about the promised *assistance.*[xvi]

"I need assistance in filing my claims. I don't understand how to identify the procedures and medical codes so I can assign the required cost when I get a global bill from the doctor. I live in the Philippines."

Response:

"Attach a readable copy of the provider's bill to the claim form, making sure it contains the following:

Sponsor's Social Security number (SSN) (eligible former spouses should use their SSN)

Provider's name and address (if more than one provider's name is on the bill, circle the name of the person who treated you)

Date and place of each service

Description of each service or supply furnished

Charge for each service

Diagnosis (if the diagnosis is not on the bill, be sure to complete block 8a on the form)

The provider you receive services from should provide you with the above information."

Some *examples*[xvii] of typical "itemized" bills from local providers.

It should be obvious that what we are told by TMA/DHA and ISOS has little basis in the reality of the local health care industry billing practices. Proof that TMA/DHA has been aware of this since

October 2013 but continue to require what they now know is impossible will be shown in the discussion on the TRICARE Philippine Demonstration Project.

At times ISOS will ask the beneficiary to go back to the provider and ask them to certify that the CPT codes are correct and that the amounts charged by procedure are normal, reasonable and customary which the provider cannot do since CPT coding is not accomplished in the Philippines by the vast majority nor do they bill by procedure. (The exception is defrauders who learned coding or were taught by ISOS but they don't really follow standard coding protocol.) When the provider declines to certify the information because he doesn't understand the codes or bill at the procedure level those procedures will be denied for payment causing the beneficiary to again pay a larger than normal share. I have personal *experience*[xviii] with this policy.

Often times when a beneficiary submits an inpatient professional fee bill that is not itemized ISOS will send them a *letter*[xix] advising them of the requirement and tell them their provider can provide the required itemized and costed bill. We already addressed above what kind of assistance TMA/DHA and ISOS will provide with obtaining this mandated information.

The reality is, TRICARE beneficiaries are required to learn medical coding and medical terminology or pay a substantial portion of your medical expenses above what others using TRICARE anywhere else in the world would pay. No other beneficiaries in the world are required to have this level of knowledge of medical coding to submit claims and it creates an incentive to use defrauders where medical coding and terminology are not needed to receive care. This possibly unintentional but now deliberate result of the implementation of the CMAC has become a major source of discontent among beneficiaries who find they pay 70% or more of the cost of their care because they don't understand the U.S. rules for coding and costing.[25] A *study*[xx] I did on a years' worth of claims data showed that for

---

[25] When TMA/DHA found that hundreds of providers quit in mass (http://www.stripes.com/news/dha-hopes-billing-fix-will-bring-back-philippine-hospitals-that-quit-pilot-project-1.251100) from their demonstration because they found they could not convert their local global bills into the complex and unique U.S. system of billing and were therefore not paid like beneficiaries are not paid, TMA/DHA no longer could hide behind their vail of ignorance. But they still insist that local providers can and will provide the detailed itemized bills that meet the U.S. system of billing.

beneficiary filed claims for inpatient professional fees, only 7% of the billed amount was allowed; the majority of claims were denied for failure to provide the required breakouts. That means that a beneficiary pays 93% plus 25% of the allowed 7%. Because of this many no longer bother to file claims as shown in our *survey*[xxi].

Given these changes in policy, that are unique only to the Philippines, can anyone blame beneficiaries for using groups that charge higher prices for care, which in turn cost TMA/DHA millions of dollars? This is what I mean when I say many policies drive beneficiaries to the defrauders who do provide the promised level of care without having to pay 50 to 100% of the cost of the care. In other words these policies greatly reduce access to care for beneficiaries in the Philippines and they seek care where they can get it without paying most of the cost themselves.

We know that TMA/DHA is well aware of many of these deficiencies since it is an open secret that they pay billed charges and from the start ignored the Philippine CMAC for care received by active duty military and their dependents unlike anywhere else in the world where everyone has the same standard. They openly admit to this in *DODIG report 2014-052*[xxii] where they also admit loss of access to care and increased beneficiary costs are an issue in the Philippines. Yet they continue to sit by and let retirees die for lack of care that they cannot afford to pay for themselves or let them pay for their own care.

Increased use of Medical Reviews on Claims

TMA/DHA refers to this process as "Prepayment Review" and claims to use it extensively. This is what *GAO*[xxiii] had to say about this process in June 2000.

"Contractors told us that of the many programs they administer, including Medicare and private plans, TRICARE is the most complicated, contributing to claims processing difficulties and high costs. For example, each of TRICARE's three options has a different array of benefits, copayments, and deductibles. Claims require different adjudication procedures, depending on which option is involved, and contractual requirements for prepayment review further complicate the process. Complexities such as these are manifested as thousands of edits in the adjudication logic of the claims processing system. These edits result in claims being "kicked out" of the system

for manual review, which extends processing time and increases administrative costs. Over half of TRICARE's claims are manually reviewed, a rate significantly higher than the industry average of 25 percent."

If you believe their claims, Prepayment Review is done on the vast majority of Philippine TRICARE claims. This is what RADM Hunter, the Deputy Director of TMA, had to say to a U.S. Senator, in January 2011, about *Prepayment Review*[xxiv] in the Philippines.

"While the TRICARE Standard health care benefit is uniform, we regrettably had to put cost control measures in place due to rampant fraud in the Philippines. ... These fraudulent activities in the Philippines have presented the greatest challenge for our Program Integrity (PI) office. TRICARE Management Activity PI placed 64 percent of all Philippine providers' and 77 percent of all Philippine beneficiaries' claims on pre-payment review. Wisconsin Physicians Service, the TRICARE Overseas claims processor, dedicated 90 percent of its resources to investigating fraud and abuse in the Philippines."

The term rampant or massive fraud in the Philippines seems to permeate almost all responses or comments from TMA/DHA as justification for their actions which have all but eliminated access to care for the majority of beneficiaries in the Philippines.

If we believe the statistics then we have to believe that TMA/DHA believes that a huge majority of Philippine hospitals, physicians and pharmacies are defrauders and one would assume they have some proof of that.

In the case of beneficiaries it appears the vast majority are considered defrauders as well, if you care to believe the Director. To put the 77% into prospective that means that out of ten beneficiaries made up of military retirees, their wives and kids, 8 out of 10 are attempting to defraud TRICARE. Seventy seven percent of 11,000 translates into 8,470. Considering that DOD Actuary says that there are around 4,000 military retirees one could also conclude that all 4,000 are considered defrauders as well as 4,470 of their wives and children. One can only wonder what it is in the Philippines that turns so many previously honorable and dedicated military retirees to a life of crime; maybe something in the water.

The claim that WPS expends 90% of their total resources means they only spend 10% of their time is used processing claims from around the world.

All of this is in direct contradiction to what Mr. Daniel Boucek, Special Agent in Charge, Defense Criminal Investigative Service, DoD told me in a telephone conversation not to many years ago. He said he spent more time in the Philippines investigating fraud than any other investigator. He further said that senior staff at TMA/DHA refused his invitation to come and see for themselves what the problems were. He said he didn't see fraud in the Philippines medical industry to be much different than anywhere else where about 10% of the population is involved. That doesn't mesh well with what the Director told the Senator.

The truth is we find TMA/DHA likes to make it up as they go and we can find multiple versions of the same story floating around the internet. For example the Director's own Program Integrity office did a *presentation*[xxv] in August 2010, five months before her letter to the Senator. Their version of the "facts" are much different than those the Director presented to the Senator. Facts that were used to justify to the Senator why a huge loss to access to care were unavoidable.

C&CS Communications & Customer Service Conference

PROGRAM INTEGRITY CHALLENGES

➤Philippines Presents Greatest Overseas Program Integrity Challenge

- 4,897 certified providers
- 1,735 Philippine providers are on pre-payment review
- 9,857 total beneficiaries.
- 2,200 Philippine beneficiaries are on pre-payment review (many as a ID theft protective measure)
- 82% of the overseas claims reviewed by TMA's Program Integrity are Philippine claims – Philippine claims make up only 16% of overseas claims
- 90% of WPS's Program Integrity's resources are dedicated to the Philippines

Many Faces, One Voice - Putting the "I Care" in TRICARE

This is slide 8 from the presentation.

Remember she said 64% of Philippine providers claims were on pre-payment review. If you calculate the percentage from the slide above it works out to 35% or close to half what the Senator was told. Recall she said 77% of beneficiary claims were on pre-payment review. Again if you do the math from above, it works out to 22%. That's less than a third of what she told the Senator. On top of that note the comment that many of those beneficiaries are on pre-payment review as a protective measure against ID theft which has absolutely nothing to do with fraud committed by the beneficiary as the Director led the Senator to believe. Finally the 90% that the Director talks about seems to be deliberately misleading as well. She infers that 90% of the claims contractors resources are taken over in fighting fraud in the Philippines where PI claims it is 90% of the contractors Program Integrity staff. I would be surprised of the WPS PI staff comprised more than 10% of the claims contractor's total staff. One sees an entirely different picture and it should become clear that the information was manipulated in order to paint as bad a picture as possible to make the point the Director was trying to make and mislead the Senator so he would not pursue the issues addressed to him and to place the writer in as bad a light as possible.

Over the last ten years I have seen many examples of this in newspaper articles and various presentations TMA/DHA made to beneficiaries and service organizations. The latest example is Lt. Gen Robb's response to the House Armed Services Committee. It appears to be a concerted effort to justify their draconian approaches and ward off investigations into the sever loss of access to care afforded TRICARE beneficiaries in the Philippines.

Prepayment review slows down the processing of claims and can require additional information and justification before paying a claim. Two examples of what we know have been demanded in the past.

- Double proof that the amount paid to the provider was actually paid. This includes such things as proving that the patient had money in bank accounts and withdraws of sufficient amounts on or shortly before the actual payment of the bills. Other documents might consist of credit card statements or loan documents.
- Detailed narratives from the provider justifying the procedures, intensity of care and billed amounts.

Impact of These Actions

Each year the TMA/DHA Program Integrity office publishes an end of year report. In it they detail the dollar savings from the various programs implemented overseas, most of which were implemented uniquely in the Philippines.

A typical analysis of the program and its impact was addressed in the 2007 report which we extracted below.

"A large number of overseas providers, particularly in the Philippines, have been placed on prepayment review. This has resulted in disallowed services that otherwise would have been paid had these providers suspected of billing the program inappropriately not been placed on prepayment review. The reported savings captured from prepayment review of overseas providers for calendar year 2007 was $3,357,472.

In addition to prepayment review of providers, some overseas beneficiaries have been placed on prepayment review status. The reported savings captured from prepayment review of overseas beneficiary claims for calendar year 2007 was $617,496. The overseas screening of claims also led to claim denials of $13,493,543 for calendar year 2007."

From 2006 until 2007 they broke out the three categories of savings. As they indicated in 2006 and 2007 the biggest contributor to these savings was the Philippines. We briefly discussed what prepayment review was and in 2007 they said that they saved through denial of payment of claims $3,357,472 from providers and $617,496 from beneficiaries. The other area, screening of claims garnered them the major share of what they tote as savings, $13,493,543. From information we gained from discussions with various TMA/DHA employees the screening of claims denials are claims denied because providers were not certified or amounts disallowed because they exceeded the CMAC or because the beneficiary or provider were not versed enough in the U.S. medical coding and claims filing rules and processes to convert local global bills to the unique U.S. itemized and costed system.

As can clearly been seen the vast majority of their savings came from programs that were poorly designed and much of their claimed savings come on the backs of beneficiaries. Starting in 2008 they no longer broke out the savings from denied claims into the categories.

This chart depicts the amounts claimed as Cost Avoidance by year. While it includes all of overseas, based on PI comments, the majority of this savings came from the Philippines.

Cost Avoidance Due to Program Integrity Actions	
Year	Amount Claimed
2006	$9,079,611
2007	$17,468,511
2008	$20,813,073
2009	$31,411,320
2010	$11,497,249
2011	$791,041
2012	$3,507,750
2013	$4,222,166

The graph, below, is a graphical depiction of the same information.

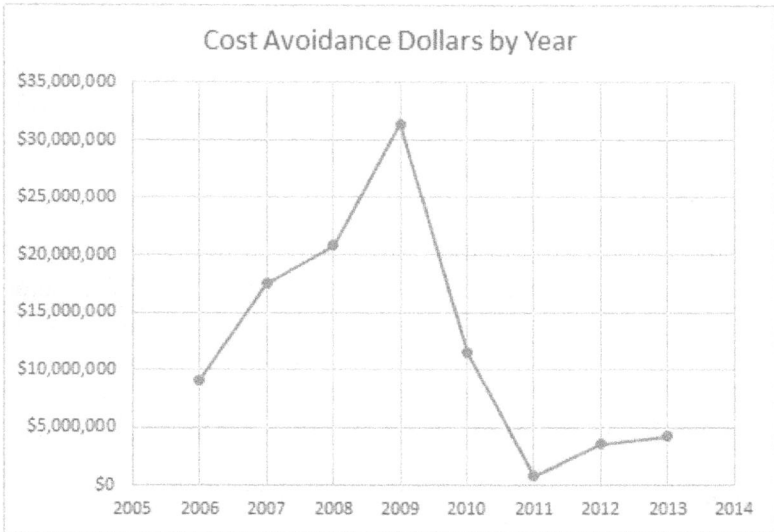

Cost Avoidance Dollars by Year

There was a significant drop in these dollars in 2011. I think that can be attributed to a combination of errors on the part of TMA/DHA or the new TOP contractor, ISOS, since they were not listed for 2011 but had the contract. The long term trend from 2010 forward is a significant drop in these cost avoidance dollars which were primarily made up of denials of claims involving certification and the CMAC.

What happened between 2009 and 2011 to cause the dramatic drop? There are two things we are aware of that would have had a dramatic impact in this area. First in the 2009 timeframe a major hospital in Manila, The Medical City (TMC), decided it would accept TRICARE Standard beneficiaries, collect their copay and file claims. That didn't work out to well for them as they were not versed in the intricacies of the complex U.S. claims filing system nor did they have an appreciation of the impact of the CMAC and its understated fees. I have a good knowledge of this since I was hospitalized a number of times at TMC during this time and observed how they managed the claims as well as having numerous discussions with their staff. When they quite they claimed they had lost many millions of dollars to TRICARE and doctors associated with the hospital also lost millions of dollars in denied or unfiled claims. To give you one small example I was an inpatient 3 times during this time and all claims were denied except for one of the stays for the hospital portion. So I volunteered to refile the claims for them and ultimately they were all paid. But for thousands of inpatient and outpatient claims they were never reimbursed or reimbursed at rates much lower than the normal and customary fees for the area. So when they stopped filing claims, there were much fewer claims to deny or underpay so fewer dollars to claim as cost avoidance.

The other process that was also at work during this same time was a gradual reduction in claims filed by beneficiaries. They, like TMC discovered, could not comply with the complex demands of converting bills by medically coding and extracting individual medical procedures accomplished on them. So fewer and fewer bothered to file claims; why spend money on copying documents and postage when you got nothing in return. A secondary cause was underpayment of legitimate claims due to the CMAC that was not properly designed for the Philippines and finally claims denied when the beneficiary was told the provider could not be certified or did not exist. Two studies I did dramatically demonstrate this. One was a *review*[xxvi] of 2009 claims data that demonstrated that only 7% of the billed amounts for beneficiary filed claims for inpatient professional fees was allowed. The second was the *study*[xxvii], using 2010 data, showing that reimbursement rates in the Philippines after adjustments for cost differences was only 13% of what TMA/DHA spent on beneficiaries anywhere else in the world.

Creation of a Network

To quote from The Journal of Public Inquiry, Fall/Winter 2005, *TRICARE OVERSEAS PROGRAM (TOP) FRAUD*[xxviii], by Daniel M. Boucek.

"During the years TOP has existed, TMA has been cautious about making changes. With that in mind, the recommendation is for incremental changes leading to a network of certified providers. Using a provider network automatically puts in place controls that do not exist under TOP as it exists today. Most importantly, the costs for services will be regulated. The new policy would likely mirror, to the extent possible, existing healthcare programs in the United States. One option for TMA consideration may include a partnership with Blue Cross Philippines, which has a network of approved providers operating under a reasonable cost schedule."

As we know from the article TMA/DHA resists change and in particular change from the outside. We also know from this article and discussions with Mr. Boucek that those outside TMA/DHA saw the ultimate solution to fraud and access to care as the implementation of a locally contracted provider network. The use of this vehicle would provide for a nationwide network of providers with a local reasonable cost schedule. This was the vision and hope for the ultimate solution.

A PPO, properly implemented, would allow TMA/DHA to eliminate provider certification at a savings of hundreds of thousands of dollars a year and eliminate most claims processing at a savings of millions and negotiate a discount on care also saving additional money as well as the savings from the elimination of fraud. The side benefit would be a more accessible benefit for beneficiaries where they only had to pay their co-pay at time of care which would be less due to negotiated discounts in the cost of care and not using defrauders which charge more. In fact it is reasonable to expect a savings in the neighborhood of millions a year, primarily through lower contract costs, if this was applied. This is a win-win situation for all concerned so it is hard to understand TMA/DHA's reluctance to move forward with this.[26]

---

[26] To develop my estimated savings I used information extracted from DODIG reports and information supplied at various times by TMA/DHA either through emails, letters or information available to bidders for the recent TOP contract. I also conducted interviews with PPOs. The mentioned Blue Cross didn't seem to have a plan that would mesh with

Most of the fraud and the limited access to care could be rectified by replacing the Philippine unique policies with a local contract PPO as was agreed to long ago with the benefits that were outlined in the above article. MG Granger agreed with my assessment of implementing a capitated PPO and indicated a desire to implement it in the Philippines as a pilot program before considering propagating it too much of the rest of the world where sufficient beneficiaries resided. However, by the time he saw the benefit, he was close to retirement and apparently wasn't able to carry it forward.

The Real Data

That brings us to the TMA/DHA built replacement for the agreed to local PPO that goes by the name, TRICARE Demonstration Project for the Philippines but commonly called the Demo. We first became aware of the Demo in September 2011 when one of our members discovered a short notice announcing it in the *Federal Register*[xxix]. However, TMA/DHA made no effort to inform Philippine beneficiaries of the project or had they discussed it with beneficiaries prior to the notice in the Federal Register to get their input or concerns about more changes to their already limited TRICARE Standard benefit; changes that affect nobody else in the world but them.

TMA/DHA has no assets on the ground and nobody with a knowledge of the Philippine health care industry. When we heard about this we attempted to offer our assistance; we were rejected out of hand. At the time my group offered to assist and contacted RADM

TRICARE while another, Kanios Health Management, seemed much more progressive and willing to accommodate. In fact we obtained a proposed health plan and price quotes for a policy to cover the majority of care for retirees and their families from them which at the time was being considered because many retirees felt their benefit would cease to exist when the original 22.9% was going to be applied to the CMAC. The reality is that the price quoted to me in a formal proposal was quite reasonable and demonstrates that a properly managed capitated PPO could save millions. As I'm sure you already know by using a capitated PPO, with a reinsurance provision, would incentivize the contractor to eliminate fraud and negotiate discounts as these actions would insure their profit and result in savings to the taxpayer. This, balanced with an on the ground TMA/DHA employee to insure access to care is maintained provides the best solution for both cost savings and access. I was able to show that there would be a substantial saving in the cost of care in the Philippines. Because I didn't have access to all the data I would have liked, my cost saving estimates were conservative. However I believe that the potential for legitimate savings is achievable using this approach instead of savings on the backs of beneficiaries.

Hunter, the Deputy Director of TMA at the time. We asked for specific information on how it was planned to be implemented so we could offer cautions and suggestions. She said she would direct CAPT Rothacker, the Director of TAO-P, to provide the requested information. After waiting some time without any contact we attempted to contact CAPT Rothacker. For weeks our emails were ignored. Finally he responded claiming his email system, @med.navy.mil, had been down so he did not receive our emails. He asked for some time to respond. More weeks passed without a response which prompted a new inquiry. Finally we got the truth from him as he responded that he was not able to provide any information per the guidance he received since the program had not been finalized yet. Bottom line, after the weeks of run-a-round we were completely shut out.[27]

In late November 2011 the Stars and Stripes (S&S), with our input, did an extensive *article*[xxx] on the issues we face in the Philippines. In an interview with TMA/DHA they told S&S that the project was scheduled for implementation in the spring of 2012 and that in the coming months they would hire a contractor. A couple of weeks later we discovered that in fact the contractor had been hired well before the interview with S&S and was ISOS. In April 2012, when we met with TMA/DHA and their contract staff, we were informed that the program had been delayed but no new time was set nor were any reasons given. Later an update to the TRICARE Operations Manual indicated a start date of 1 January 2013. We would later find that one of the major reasons for the delay was the inability of ISOS to recruit providers who would agree to the provisions of the Demo which TMA/DHA also alluded to in their recent response to the DODIG.

Before we go further let's look at what TMA/DHA claims in the Federal Register notice, a portion of which is extracted below. Of note is the areas in bold.

---

[27] TMA/DHA would later publicly claim that they sought and obtained input from a number of beneficiaries. In a statement in a Stars & Stripes article (http://www.stripes.com/news/pacific/philippines/retirees-still-to-face-upfront-medical-payments-in-philippines-1.197918) they said, "It [TRICARE] said this month it has built plans based on input from the military beneficiaries." To date, I have not found one beneficiary that claims to have provided input, not one. This included more than 400 on our forum, a few thousand that read our Newsletters and questions posed at RAO Manila meetings. Once again this appears to be one of those unsubstantiated "truths" that TMA/DHA puts out.

"TRICARE has experienced dramatic increases in the amount billed for healthcare services rendered in the Philippines from $15 million in 1999 to $59 million in 2009 while the number of beneficiaries has remained constant. Administrative controls such as the validation of providers, implementation of a fee reimbursement schedule, duplicate claims edits and the impact of the cost-shares and deductibles have limited actual TRICARE expenditures to $17 million in 2009 for only approximately 11,000 beneficiaries.

In addition to these administrative controls, fraud and abuse activities in the Philippines have been a growing concern that necessitated prompt investigation and actions to reduce the number of fraudulent or abusive incidences. Measures were taken to prevent or reduce the level of fraud and abuse against TRICARE while concurrent investigations and prosecutions were conducted. In April 2008, seventeen individuals were convicted of defrauding the TRICARE program of more than $100 million.

*As a result, prepayment review of claims is conducted to identify excessive charges and aberrant practices. Prepayment review is a tool typically used on a limited basis. **Nevertheless, these efforts alone are not expected to control and eliminate the rising costs in the Philippines."***

The obvious intent of this information from the notice is to convince us that there is still a significant fraud problem in the Philippines and all their efforts have not been sufficient. Therefore these additional controls and reduced access to care policies are necessary. Let's look at what and how they claim this. The first obvious issue is the claim that the number of beneficiaries remained constant between 1999 and 2009. The *DOD Actuary*[xxxi] maintains data on the number of military retirees and survivors by country. While we were not able to obtain their data for 1999 or 2000, we do have it from 2001 through 2013. See the chart to the right. Every year between 2001 and 2013 has shown a steady increase in the population. Even if we assume 1999 and 2000 are anomalies and had no growth there was still a documented growth of almost 10% between the dates TMA/DHA claims there was none. It seems obvious they claim this hoping to garner additional support for their position. To calculate total beneficiary population we generally use a factor of 1.69 dependents per sponsor (retiree and survivor).

DOD Actuary Retiree & Survivor Population	
2001	3,727
2009	4,088
Increase	361
Percent Increase	9.69%

In August 2011, about two months before TMA/DHA posted the notice, they and WPS conducted a meeting in Manila for a limited number of retirees. Among the *presentations*[xxxii] was one that showed claims filed, billed and paid amounts by year.

Using billed, instead of paid amounts appears to be another attempt to garner additional support. It is well known that *billed amounts*[xxxiii] are commonly inflated which are not paid by insurance companies including in the U.S. While the $15 million for 1999 matches what was presented in Manila, the $59 million for 2009 is confusing since it doesn't even come close to what was presented two months earlier which is $82 million for 2009.

If paid amounts were used the story would look much different, $10 million in 1999 to $27 million in 2013. We know their claim that there was no increase in beneficiaries and we know that was wrong. We also know that in a real analysis inflation needs to be considered. Below is the annual consumer price inflation rates for the period in question taken from the *World Bank*[xxxiv].

Year	1999	2000	2001	2002	2003	2004	2005	2006	2007	2008	2009	Total
Annual Inflation	5.9%	4.0%	5.3%	2.7%	2.3%	4.8%	6.5%	5.5%	2.9%	8.3%	4.2%	52.4%
Taken from the World Bank annual consumer price inflation by country												

The claim that they limited expenditures, paid amounts, to $17 million is way off as well by about $10 million when compared with the data presented in Manila two months earlier.

If these factors were taken into consideration and paid amounts compared the case would have been much weaker. The really troubling aspect of their claims and narrative is that, while they knew the billed and paid amounts for 2010 when they published this information they chose to leave them out. It becomes obvious why they left them out once you see them; billed amount $33.3 million and paid amount $8.3 million. If they had included them then their final conclusion, *"Nevertheless, these efforts alone are not expected to control and eliminate the rising costs in the Philippines."* would have been false. In fact they would have had to admit that their current limitations, provider certification, CMAC and prepayment review had reduced access to care to a point where almost nobody was obtaining care where TRICARE paid their fair share. Using 2010 data that TMA/DHA included in their annual report to congress and publicly available from Medicare we showed that in 2010 that TMA/DHA expended just 13% of what would have been expected per beneficiary in the Philippines as compared to the rest of the world. Using current data would have made it extremely difficult for them to justify continued use of the current measures while adding the additional restrictions imposed under the Demo.

If we take the paid amounts for 1999 and 2009 as presented in Manila and then extrapolate the expected paid amount considering population change and inflation over the ten years it is easy to see just how bad access to care is in the Philippines.

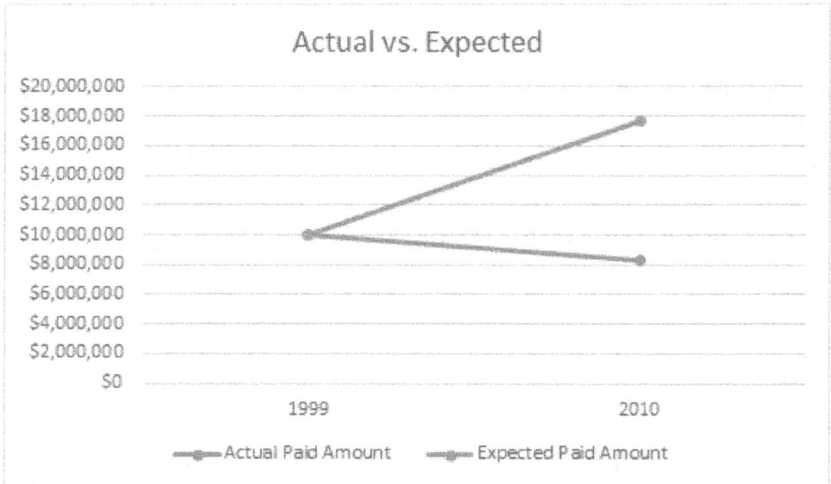

Demo Policy Changes

In addition to a new start date an update to the TRICARE Operations Manual provided us with a little more specific information on the Demo. One policy that was made clearer was it was likely that a significant amount of care would be under the alternate limited

Philippine TRICARE Standard rules; rules that required the patient pay in advance and file claims.

The expanded explanation is addressed at paragraph 4.9 of the revision to the *TRICARE Operations Manual*[xxxv]. Essentially what it says is in the event they cannot recruit sufficient providers who will agree to the requirements they will add providers called "Certified Providers" who beneficiaries will be required to see. However these providers will require cash payment at time of care and the beneficiary will then have to file a claim. Essentially they will be required to use the same system in use now but without the current choice of providers everyone else on Standard has. These claims will be subject to the same policies and practices imposed on us now and result in beneficiaries once again having to pay for the majority of their care but under a new program entitled the Demo. In practice more than 60% of all specialties would fall under this exception.

Once the program got underway we were to find that there were many changes and exceptions added by TMA/DHA and ISOS in an attempt to keep the program going.

1. Reversal on payment of deductibles and copays

One of the hallmarks of the Demo was that beneficiaries would not have to pay upfront and that providers would file claims and collect deductibles and copays after the claim was adjudicated. This was the first major policy to fall and was done because ISOS discovered that local providers were not willing to sign up under these rules. So the policy was arbitrarily changed and TMA/DHA attempted to justify the change claiming it was the idea of beneficiaries. I was at the meeting in Manila with 8 other retirees where this was brought up as an option requesting input. While one individual indicated one positive reason for the change the rest voiced various concerns and after a few minutes of discussion ISOS moved to another subject. Stars & Stripes published an *article*[xxxvi] on this major change.

When I questioned senior management at ISOS about what safeguards were in place to insure that the providers would file claims they initially begged the question and finally told me that it was none of our business as what was in the agreements was proprietary. What I know is there is no mandated requirement that they file claims. TMA/DHA assumed that they would file claims in order to be paid. They removed that incentive by requiring beneficiary upfront payments of deductibles and the providers see no reason to spend money filing claims that bring them nothing in return. Both ISOS and TMA/DHA know this but have done nothing to correct their mistake.

Multiple Demo hospitals have advised beneficiaries that they have no intention of filing claims when the full cost of the care is covered by deductibles or in one instance only after all of "their" claims are filed. To our knowledge after surveying hundreds of retirees only one has seen an EOB and received credit for their deductible. Some have over paid their deductible and have never received a refund as promised by TMA/DHA. In addition many found that promised copay refunds never came and calls to ISOS result in being told to go chase the provider which we were told would not happen.

2. Medical supply and out of stock items the hospital doesn't want to purchase

This is an example of a policy that ISOS agreed to with hospitals but saw no need to inform beneficiaries. We have no idea if they bothered to inform TMA/DHA. I first became aware of this issue when a beneficiary informed me that he was required to pay for multiple supply items during his hospitalization in violation of the published policy. My initial inquiry to ISOS met with a non-answer and further inquiries were ignored. I then contacted TMA/DHA and eventually the new policy was published that says hospitals can require that Demo patients pay cash for medical supply items and equipment. One Demo hospital requires patients pay for all medical supplies, pharmacy etc. at time of care. In some cases this can result in thousands of dollars that have to be paid up front. In all cases the beneficiary is required to file a claim.

3. Lens required for cataract surgery

We were not so lucky with this secretly negotiated policy by ISOS. When I went for cataract surgery I was advised by the physician that lenses were not a TRICARE benefit and I would have to purchase it myself. This is far from the truth and I questioned him on this. He informed me that he was told this by the ISOS trainer, although he wasn't aware they were ISOS trainers. He said a local company Global 24 had designed a "new" TRICARE program for the Philippines and all the old players were gone. He went on to say they said filing claims was simple and would be paid and paid within 30 days unlike the "old" TRICARE that owed him thousands of dollars. He said that the trainer told him he could charge beneficiaries for lenses as they were not part of the TRICARE benefit. He was upset when I told him Global 24 had no local offices and was owned by ISOS; one of the old players.

My initial contact with ISOS resulted in being told it should be covered and the physician was making up the story. Using other beneficiaries I was able to determine that all the Ophthalmologists at two separate hospitals in two separate Demo areas had the identical policy. I reported this to TMA/DHA suggesting that ISOS be required to retrain the providers. This was agreed to and a few weeks later I was informed that the training was being conducted. Seven months later I went back for cataract surgery in my other eye and to my surprise I was again informed that the lens was not part of the benefit and I would have to pay; the physician told me nobody from ISOS ever spoke to him about it since we spoke before. I inquired with the hospital staff about the policy and was told they had specific guidance that charging the beneficiary was allowed under the Demo and they provided the name of the ISOS employee. I then emailed and called ISOS to complain that again I was required to pay. I was told by the person on the phone that she didn't know what to do but would pass the issue up and promised I would have an answer by the next day; it's been almost year and I'm still waiting for their response. I ended up paying once again in violation of published policy. Another inquiry to TMA/DHA resulted in ISOS finally admitting they had negotiated a secret policy with Ophthalmologists that allowed them to require beneficiaries pay cash for the lenses. I suggested that they should at least publicize this previously secret policy but was told TMA/DHA saw no reason to do that. So I publicized it as best I could through my group's blog and newsletter.

Demo Location Disappears Without a Word

When we were finally told where the Demo would take place it became obvious that TMA/DHA and ISOS had little idea where the beneficiary population centers are located. We were told there would be three phases. Phase I would include Metro Manila, Angeles City, Olongapo City and Orion, Bataan. Phase II would include General Trias, Naic, Bacoor and Imus, Cavite and Cavite City. Phase III would include Iloilo City.

We were also told that once Phase III was in place that the majority of beneficiaries would be covered. Our best estimates of where beneficiaries reside leaves about 40% outside these areas which represent about 2% of the physical Philippines.

Nobody could understand how Orion, Bataan got in the mix. Orion is a second class municipality with a population of around 50,000 and is rather isolated with no major public transportation in and out; people have to first take local transportation to the provincial capital, Balanga City. What my group discovered was that there were few medical providers in the area and one hospital. We also found that there were maybe a dozen TRICARE beneficiaries in the area and most lived in Balanga but TMA/DHA and ISOS didn't know this. Claims came from one of those providers that were certified under questionable conditions and who then submitted claims, many probably fraudulently. Since TMA/DHA used claims submissions as a proxy to determine population size and location this little town popped up on the radar. When this was brought to TMA/DHA's attention they immediately and quietly removed Orion from the Demo and have refused to explain how they could have made such a mistake.

Mass Resignation from the Demo

A major *failure*[xxxvii] of the program occurred in October 2013, just ten months into the Demo. The area affected, which includes the single largest beneficiary population in the Philippines, has still not recovered. They have but one hospital which most do not consider the best hospital in the area and just 32 physicians; much of the care is obtained using the limited TRICARE Standard plan due to waivers and lack of qualified providers. In that month all hospitals and providers quit in mass because they were not paid because they did not understand the unique requirements that are required to convert local global bills to detailed listings of procedures with costs broken out to match the CMAC rates. Most that received a few payments also found they were generally underpaid based on local customary rates. ISOS had onsite employees at the hospitals but apparently they, ISOS and TMA/DHA didn't have a clue what was going to happen because for a week after the resignations all were silent and wouldn't even respond to questions from Stars & Stripes. Eventually they responded to Stars & Stripes but not to beneficiaries. The *promised fix*[xxxviii] as described by TMA/DHA was not successful in recruiting sufficient replacements. For one the attitude of TMA/DHA that the problem is the fault of providers who failed to properly document their billings goes a long way in showing how well they work with overseas providers. The other claim that ISOS put *"claims liaison officers in the Philippines to help the providers with properly filing claims and avoiding delays"* has proven to be bogus and if it was true would expose them to sever conflict of interest charges.

My interaction with numerous physicians in Angeles City indicated most had no intention of returning. In addition my conversations with Demo providers in Manila indicate they are just as unhappy and some are already quitting the Demo but on an individual basis; mass resignations may follow later. Some Demo physicians found that I successfully process claims for beneficiaries and also assisted The Medical City with a number of claims in the past. One has text and emailed me requesting assistance in processing and reprocessing his claims so he can get at least some reimbursement. I informed him not to expect full reimbursement because of the CMAC understatement of local rates in surgical procedures but he should see some improvement in his reimbursements. Since he is resigning from the Demo, which will limit the number of claims, I agreed to assist him as well. I do this without reimbursement but as one individual cannot possibly assist in conversion on all claims for more than 11,000 beneficiaries.

Population Served

TMA/DHA claims that 72% of TRICARE beneficiaries live within 100 miles of Metro Manila and the balance, 28%, live in the provinces beyond and based on 10 year old data. That means that approximately 7,920 live within 100 miles of Metro Manila and 3,080 live in the provinces beyond. See the first page of their *chart*[xxxix].

When the Demo is fully implemented Angeles City, Olongapo City, Metro Manila, parts of Cavite province and Iloilo City will constitute the entire area serviced by the Demo; at least for limited care that doesn't meet one of the exceptions. Even if these figures were correct, why would anyone believe that the majority of the 7,920 live only in these first four limited locations when there are hundreds of others to choose from? And further that the majority of those living in the provinces beyond, 3,080, live in a single city, Iloilo City? If we consider 95% as being who is covered that means all beneficiaries within the 100 mile radius of Manila live within one of the first four areas except 396. That means all those living northeast of Manila to a point just south of Dugupan or southwest a little past Lucena and east in Bataan are no more than 396 total. Once Iloilo City in the provinces is added only another 154 beneficiaries will be excluded including those that live in Baguio, San Fernando La Union, Naga City, Cebu City, CDO, Tacloban, Davao and dozens more locations. To add further controversy when viewing the *chart*[xl] look at the figures on the second page and compare their figures for retirees in the Western Pacific compared to the official figures from the *DOD Actuary*[xli]. If they can't even get these basic figures right, what chance is there that the calculations on the first page and used for the Demo have any validity? The only people that would believe that are those that have no understanding of where people live in the Philippines and have spent no time here.

As we can see a proxy using historical claims submissions has flaws. Our *survey*[xlii] of retirees in the Philippines indicate that 76% do not file claims but pay for their own care. That means that most beneficiaries don't file claims. So who filed the claims used to determine where beneficiaries lived? The answer is providers that were operating in a few areas using the practices invented by HVC and certified even though they did meet the basic requirements for certification.[28] These providers submitted the majority of the claims. Although I *reported*[xliii] these certifications that allowed these groups to function as physician groups without any real physicians and physicians to bill as hospitals, TMA/DHA ignored the problem for years. Once one understands who filed claims and who did not, it becomes clear any attempt to convert claim volume into beneficiary

---

[28] These certifications are discussed earlier in section, The Consequences Resulting From the TMA/DHA Modifications to the Philippine Benefit.

location is flawed. The glaring example of how flawed the conclusions are is when they programmed Orion, Bataan as one of the Phase I sites and was included right up to the last minute until it was brought to their attention by us and then quietly removed.

If we are going to use a proxy I prefer to use another one and one that probably better demonstrates the actual distribution of the TRICARE population. The proxy is where HVC placed its clinics and hospitals. Since they were in the business of filing inflated claims for care provided TRICARE beneficiaries it only makes sense they placed their facilities where there were large enough populations to make it worth their while. We also know that HVC paid finders to go out and locate TRICARE beneficiaries, many of whom are Filipino-Americans and survivors and their children but it is unlikely TMA/DHA and ISOS are aware of this. A few years back TMA/DHA conveniently produced a slide presentation with a *map*[xliv] of the Philippines that pinpointed the locations of all the HVC facilities. Using this we can produce a list of cities where the beneficiary population lived in sufficient numbers to make it worthwhile for HVC to invest in facilities and staff to treat and file claims on them. If one matches some older Certified Provider lists, before access to care was reduced and beneficiaries stopped filing claims, the number of certified providers in these areas can be used as a second proxy to determine the relative size of the beneficiary population in some of these locations.

First review the *map*[xlv] and then the beneficiary *population estimates*[xlvi] based on the two proxies. It is clear that the Demo will not cover a significant number of beneficiaries and even where it is physically implemented it only covers them part time as there are as many exceptions to the rules as there are rules. Further those that reside within the 2% of the Philippines covered by the Demo will not be covered when they step outside these small geographic locations. For example a beneficiary living in Angeles City decides to drive to Manila; both areas are Demo areas. During the hour on the road between these two areas, if they have an accident and need medical care they are again on their own. They will have to pay for their care and take their chances on getting reimbursed in a system that fails to reimburse for most care.

Quality of providers

Under Overseas TRICARE Standard a beneficiary is able to choose any legitimate provider, thereby transferring the responsibility of determining the quality of providers to the beneficiary; the same as Standard in the states.

Early on TMA/DHA limited this access for Philippine TRICARE with their certified provider requirement. But the limitation was minimal as only a few providers refused certification although it appears refusals have been increasing in recent years as more honest providers are adversely affected by TMA/DHA policies.

With the advent of the Demo TMA/DHA severely restricted access to a limited number of providers and in many cases a single provider, much like Prime. Except Prime does quality checks on providers and it is a voluntary program where the Demo is mandatory and has no quality checks. To opt out of the Demo results in the beneficiary paying for 100% of the cost of their care. Beneficiaries living outside Demo areas that were never taught the rules suffer the same fate if they happen to obtain care within a Demo area.

When TMA/DHA first published their intent to implement this mandatory program in the *Federal Register*[xlvii] they said;

"...while ensuring beneficiaries have sufficient access to high quality care."

Then again in the TRICARE Operations Manual 6010.56-M, Chapter 18, Section 12, para 1.0 they said,

"...while providing high quality, safe health care to TRICARE Standard beneficiaries residing in the Philippines and receiving care in designated demonstration area(s)."

Then in para 5.2.5 they said,

"Provide certification oversight and monitor quality of care for providers and institutional facilities as prescribed in Chapter 24, Section 4; 32 CFR 199.6; and TPM, Chapter 12."

I already knew that there were no real quality checks done on Demo providers but tried to address it with both ISOS and TMA/DHA. At the first limited attendance (9 retirees) meeting held by ISOS in Manila shortly before the Demo started I questioned Mr. Frewen, Vice President Operations TRICARE Asia Pacific ISOS about what quality checks were done on Demo providers. He responded by saying that only certified providers would be considered to be Demo providers. Since all Demo providers had to be certified first that obviously was a non-answer. I pointed out to him that I knew that the TOM didn't require any quality checks on overseas providers. He then said that by using certified providers they would be using only providers that beneficiaries had used before, thereby insuring only quality providers were used. While obliquely this might have some limited truth, the reality is a beneficiary may see whatever provider is available but nobody sees them again, or as in my case seeing a provider only to discover that they had not attended Continuing Medical Education for years and so never saw them again. I also found, as the Demo progressed, they brought on providers that no beneficiary had ever seen before and this was shown when we monitored them on the lists. The provider would appear as a newly certified provider and also as an approved provider at the same time or the following month. Obviously this violated Mr. Frewen's quality check process.

Later we posed the same question in writing to ISOS and received the typical non-answer; again "begging the question". So we went back in great detail and explained quality standards, how they are applied in the states and specifically asked.

"Given your comment below please provide the specific reviews that are conducted. Please be specific and list each item and area reviewed including the expected standards providers are required to meet. If standards are applied due to membership, such as JCI or a local association, please provide a link to their specific standards. Since requirements for hospitals and physicians should be significantly different, please provide two lists, one for hospitals and one for physicians."

I got yet another answer but again they declined to provide the information requested. Instead they attempted to imply quality checks were done.

"Providers selected for the Demonstration Project have undergone quality and credentialing checks in line with the requirements of the TRICARE Overseas Program. It has been clearly defined at all stages that the Approved Providers have also met all requirements to be certified providers."

Obviously this is begging the question once again because, if they answered honestly, they would have to admit there are essentially no quality checks. If there were I know they would be the first to point them out by answering the specific questions I asked.

If one reads through the TRICARE Overseas Program (TOP) requirements one will find references to quality checks and if one reads through the requirements for Certification of Philippine providers one will find the same references. However, if one reads further through the TRICARE Operations Manual 6010.56-M *Chapter 24, Section 4*[xlviii], Host Nation Providers, one will find the following.

"2.1 The TOP contractor will be responsible for provider certification oversight, and monitoring of provider/institution quality. The contractor shall use Chapter 4, 32 CFR 199.6, and TPM, Chapter 11 to the maximum extent possible for the certification of host nation providers. The contractor is not required to follow TRICARE requirements for United States (U.S.) credentialing standards [quality checks], except that services that are specifically linked to the Medicare program..."

What this says is the TOP contractor is exempt from the quality standards when the provider is not part of the Medicare program. Since Medicare does not apply in the Philippines they have no requirement to do quality checks; they do insist they are licensed and meet some administrative requirements on a checklist. But they would prefer you not know that because then we would know that TMA/DHA's claim *"You will have access to providers who deliver high-quality medical care."* is completely bogus.

So what are the real requirements to become an Approved Provider? The obvious answer, beyond being licensed by the government, is there are only administrative requirements. They have to sign a secret agreement, which Mr. Frewen claims the contents of which are none of our business.[29] Essentially they have to show a willingness to collect deductibles and copays and acknowledge they know they can submit claims if they want and perhaps be willing to increase fees for Demo patients. They also have to acknowledge that they understand the provisions of 32 CFR, Part 199.9 which includes this provision.

"199.9 (b) (2) Improper billing practices. Examples include, charging CHAMPUS beneficiaries rates for services and supplies that

---

[29] When I questioned what provisions were in these agreements that would insure that providers file claims when the entire cost of care was already paid because of deductibles he told me the agreements are proprietary and therefore beneficiaries are not allowed to know the contents.

are in excess of those charges routinely charged by the provider to the general public, commercial health insurance carriers, or other federal health benefit entitlement programs for the same or similar services."

While ISOS tried to cover up the lack of quality checks the TMA/DHA Beneficiary Education and Support Branch was open and above board when they told us in an email that there were no requirements to do quality checks on overseas providers and in spite of what TMA/DHA and ISOS claimed.

It should be clear that Philippine beneficiaries who are required to use the Demo are limited to a small, sometimes single, selection of providers and that these providers have not undergone any commonly accepted process to determine the quality of their services. As one more example of this see this *video*[xlix] of one hospital in one Demo area that is approved and meets their "quality" standards.

Lack of Training and Official Documentation on the Demonstration

During the last week of October 2012 TMA/DHA and ISOS conducted three training sessions on the Demo. Notice of the meetings was about a week in advance of the meetings and the meetings were limited in size and TMA/DHA allowed only selected beneficiaries to attend. I attended the meeting in Manila where there were 9 participants. Across all three meetings less than 50 military retirees attended. The number of attendants were limited due to a fear on the part of TMA/DHA and ISOS that harm may come to the presenters by angry TRICARE beneficiaries. Prior to scheduling the meetings there was a discussion with the Marine detachment at the embassy requesting assistance to protect the presenters. In the end their request was denied, resulting in sever limits placed on attendees. I know this because in the email sent to me telling me about the meetings they included the thread of emails with this discussion. I was also previously told of this fear by TMA/DHA employees. We were told these meetings with fewer than 50 beneficiaries present out of 11,000 that were affected by the Demo constituted all the Demo training that would be given.

According to the Federal Register announcing the demonstration, it stated, *"The Government, in conjunction with the contractor, will develop and implement a communication plan to inform and educate beneficiaries about the demonstration at least 60 days before the demonstration commences."* It appeared TMA/DHA considered these three brief meetings constituted the requirement to inform and educate beneficiaries as we were almost at the 60 day point. I was informed that the expectation was that those that attended the sessions were supposed to go out and train all the other beneficiaries. This was also the total training provided prior to the start of the Demo beyond some letters sent to some beneficiaries informing them there was a Demo starting in the Philippines.

Our complaints about the all but total lack of training resulted in a second round of meetings. They were announced on a weekend giving two working days' notice to the meetings. These meetings were conducted on 9 and 10 January 2013. In spite of the short notice in total about 150 beneficiaries attended, mostly sponsors. There were many questions asked and most were not answered with straight forward responses but with generalizations or innuendos. Complaints that the single approved hospital in Angeles City was refusing to see Demo patients outside 8 to 5 M-F was mostly ignored with a comment by Mr. Frewen that we should look at the positive and not the negative. Beyond that he refused to comment. Prior to that ISOS told TMA/DHA that my complaints about this were false. Obviously he would have been laughed out of the room if he tried that at the meeting.

The training of less than 200 beneficiaries in the Demo areas was considered by TMA/DHA to have met the requirement above for Phase I. The thousands that didn't attend did without. There was no attempt to train the 40% of beneficiaries that resided outside the Demo areas but who are required to comply with Demo rules when they visit one of these areas; failure to comply results in denial of payment of all effected claims. I am aware of a number of beneficiary who lived outside these areas who were adversely affected because of this. A request to TMA/DHA that they should make an exception the first time for those living outside these areas was denied. I also talked to numerous retires living in the Demo areas who had little or no idea how it worked and two instances where they didn't even know the Demo was in affect which resulted in denied claims.

TMA/DHA and ISOS like to claim that all the information needed to comply with the Demo is on the ISOS web site. While that is partially true, there are many beneficiaries in the Philippines, particularly those in the provinces, who do not have computers or access the internet. To a lesser extent this is true even in cities. For these beneficiaries there is absolutely no information available for them. The same holds true of those with computers that have no idea there is a new TRICARE program they are required to comply with and further have no links provided to research.

Many Hospitals Refused to Accept TRICARE Demo Patients after Hours

As was briefly mentioned above Mr. Frewen ignored the question about what they were going to do about hospitals, such as Angeles University Foundation and others, which only accepted Demo patients from 8-5 M-F. Outside those hours beneficiaries found they were required to pay for their care and file a claim. I addressed this issue to TMA/DHA in numerous emails and was told by them that their contractor ISOS assured them that I had no idea what I was talking about. At one point in an email TMA/DHA suggested that maybe I just didn't know where to go to find the person at the hospital that would help me. I pointed out that when I went after hours I saw the guard at the door, the woman at the information desk, staff in admissions and in the ER who all told me to go to the business office where I was told Demo patients were only accepted 8-5 M-F. That didn't seem to help as I was again told ISOS assured them what I reported was not true. I was told that my reports on numerous hospitals that had this policy was completely false as ISOS said so. Finally after recording my conversation with an employee in the business office and offering to send it to TMA/DHA was any action taken. But that was more than a month after the Demo started and many found the Demo was not working as advertised.

Patient rights

The Defense Health Agency (DHA) published *TRICARE "Patient Rights"*[1] where they claim *"As a TRICARE beneficiary, you have rights regarding your health care and responsibilities for participating in your health care decisions." DOD Instruction 6000.14*[li] includes at Enclosure 2, "DOD Patient Bill of Rights".

What they fail to note is some or all of these "Patient Rights" do not apply to beneficiaries who are forced to use the Philippine

Demonstration. They won't publicly publish those exceptions but they exist and are enforced. *TRICARE's published Patient Rights*[lii] states,

"As a patient in the Military Health System, you have the right to: Your choice of health care providers"

and DOD Instruction 6000.14 states in Enclosure 2, DOD Patient Bill of Rights and Responsibilities, Para 1.d. that patients have the right to receive information about the providers who are providing their care including professional credentials

Both of these "rights" have been denied Demo beneficiaries.

To have a choice one must have at least two alternatives. Without two choices TMA/DHA has summarily denied this "right of choice". For more than a year into the Demo this right of choice was denied under the Demo in all locations. Inquiries to ISOS addressing this rights violation were ignored as are most customer service inquiries.

Senior staff from the TMA/DHA, Beneficiary Education and Support, Customer Service Support Branch emailed us that provider quality standards did not apply overseas and further that Demo providers were not required to discuss or reveal their credentials to beneficiaries. ISOS also confirmed that our right to this information didn't apply under the Demo as they claimed the information was secret. Given this complete lack of quality checks and the limited selection of providers in the Demo, having information on the professional credentials of Demo providers becomes extremely important. But TMA/DHA chose to deny Philippine beneficiaries this right as well.

More than a year into the Demo we finally got TMA/DHA to take limited action on specialties with a single provider. But they refused to take action on single selections of hospitals saying it was up to the contractor.

Increased Fees Directed by ISOS

Shortly after the October 2012 meeting with ISOS I predicted in an email to TMA/DHA that ISOS would revert to their old practices and advise providers to increase fees to get them to agree to the Demo. My prediction was based on feedback I received from senior staff from ISOS at the meeting plus my knowledge of their past actions involving provider group certification where they taught them how to maximize return by billing at the CMAC and well above local customary rates. As they say, "You can't teach an old dog new tricks."

By mid-January 2013 it was obvious that prices were increasing by up to 4 time's local rates. We had examples of beneficiaries paying P1,000 ($23.25) for visits from the same doctors they saw a week before for P500 ($11.63). In another example in Olongapo a retiree was required to pay P2,000 ($46.51) for a visit to a doctor that he previously paid P450 ($10.47).

My first indication of these fee increases came when a retiree related to me that he paid P1,000 for a normal P500 visit. When he questioned the doctor, he was quite open saying that the fee increases were directed by ISOS. Before long others reported the same increases with similar feedback from their providers. In one case the provider said when she indicated she didn't like the TRICARE program because of previously denied claims she said ISOS offered her higher fees if she would agree to join. So we talked to a senior employee of the hospital in Angeles who said that the increased fees were not their doing but mandated by TRICARE [ISOS] in Manila. She said if we had any questions we should address them there. Our inquiry to ISOS as usual was ignored.

I contacted TMA/DHA about this apparent fraud on the part of ISOS. Instead of investigating it themselves they reported me to ISOS and asked them to comment. The response was that I lied about talking to the employee. They claimed they spoke to the employee who denied ever speaking to me and further said the employee said they would never make that claim. Later I would go back and talk to the same senior employee but this time with another retiree with me. She not only acknowledged the previous meeting but repeatedly stated that ISOS mandated the price increases and even went as far as claiming any provider that only charged their normal rate was in violation of TRICARE policy and would have to be retrained.

In addition to claiming ISOS had no part in the increases and my claims were manufactured, TMA/DHA further claimed increases of this magnitude were normal and expected.

My question.

"When can we expect to be able to once again see providers without paying double or other increases over local normal and customary fees?"

TMA/DHA's response.

"TRICARE will reimburse health care costs based on the lesser of billed charges or the Philippine fee schedule located online at

http://www.tricare.mil/CMAC/ProcedurePricing/SearchResults.aspx.
To participate in the TRICARE Department of Defense Philippine Demonstration Project, the Institutional providers have acknowledged that they will bill at the lesser of the billed charges or CMAC rates. There may be instances in which Institutional providers are charging up to the CMAC rate because of the added time and effort they expend to submit claims and understand the TRICARE Program. This is not an uncommon practice in the Philippines (and elsewhere in the world). Patients with medical insurance will in many cases be charged a higher fee to cover the costs of the additional effort in processing the claim and recovering their invoiced amounts as the providers are accepting financial risk of getting paid the outstanding amounts as opposed to an immediate cash payment from an individual."

In essence they said that the doubling or quadruple of fees is acceptable and in fact expected. Their claim that providers can add fees to cover the effort to submit claims and understand the program and also add more fees to cover their financial risk of being paid was a new one for me.

But it does beg the question; if providers can double and quadruple fees for these reasons, isn't it logical that TMA/DHA should also accept and pay higher fees to cover these efforts and risks when a beneficiary files a claim? We posed that question to a TMA/DHA employee but received no response.

This complete turnaround seemed to be an attempt to cover themselves and their contractor's actions where they told providers to increase their fees and is a total and complete reversal of years of previous claims and even their manuals. The claim that doubling and quadrupling of fees for insured patients is a complete fabrication and the reverse holds true in the states, see *Health Care: The Cost With and Without Insurance*[liii].

Our *Policy Reversal Evidence*[liv] paper includes examples of their previous claims of fraud involving local providers who doubled their fees when filing claims and with links to support them. There are also examples where TMA/DHA repeatedly proclaimed that providers would have to agree to only charge at the lower of the usual and customary charges and the established fee schedule. This abrupt change is so extreme and fraught with problems it was hard to get my head around the consequences. Program Integrity is the office responsible for fighting fraud and has been fixated on the Philippines for years. Most of the references in the paper come from them. I can only assume that these price increases, when orchestrated by local providers is considered fraud but when orchestrated by ISOS is a legitimate practice. But the end result is the same; beneficiaries and the tax payer pay more.

Under the Philippine CMAC the two top outpatient procedure codes paid by TMA/DHA are 99213 and 99214. 99213 has a maximum allowed charge of $40.16 (P1,727) and 99214 has a maximum allowed charge of $59.37 (P2,553); 99214 is a very common procedure level for those over 65 due to multiple system issues and is the top E&M code used for Medicare outpatient visits. So any provider that charges any fee up to these amounts will be paid in full and we will be responsible for deductibles and copays. In Angeles the local normal fee is generally P500 and already high compared to similar cities. So instead of paying the historical fee of P500 TMA/DHA has sanctioned fee increases between P1,727 to P2,553 or at rates between 229% and 387% above the usual customary fee and in excess of those charges routinely charged by the provider to the general public. There is not a single local insurance company, PPO or HMO that would stay in business if they agreed to pay those kinds of rates above the usual customary rates. In fact the vast majority either get the usual customary rate or a discount off that rate. In some instances, but not common, the PPO/HMO will pay a few percentage points over the local rate but that is rare and generally in locations with limited health care services according to my previous contacts with management of various HMO's. Discussions with well-respected physicians also showed that they do not increase charges when seeing patients with local insurance.[30] Additionally if a beneficiary pays cash for a visit to these same providers they will pay P500 with a co-pay of P125. At P2,553, which TMA/DHA now says is acceptable and expected under their program a beneficiary will pay a co-pay of P638. So in reality a beneficiary is better off paying cash and not even filing a claim. In essence this policy reversal has made it cheaper for beneficiaries to pay for their own care rather than bother

---

[30] When I was in Rotary in Naga City a number of physicians were also members. Because of my background in Health Care Administration I was interested in the local health care industry practices and learned a lot from them. When these increases occurred I contacted two of them and both concurred that they granted discounts to local insurance groups.

with TRICARE at all. And I am aware of some that are doing exactly that to save money.

This also is a complete and total reversal of their posted Federal Register notice.

They historically had major issues with providers that charged them higher rates than they charged locals or substantially in excess of customary or reasonable charges.

In the Federal Register notice they promised.

"To be included on the approved list, a provider must agree to accept reimbursement at the lower of the usual and customary charges and the established fee schedule."

They claimed one of the primary goals of the Demo was to control costs. Obviously that was thrown out the window when ISOS used the carrot of higher fees to get providers to join the Demo.

"The purpose of this demonstration is to validate an alternative approach to providing healthcare services for those beneficiaries covered under the TRICARE Standard option in the Philippines, controlling costs, eliminating any balance billing issues, and ensuring that the billing practices comply with regulatory requirements."

If you read through the *Policy Reversal Evidence*[lv] paper you will also see that in many instances hospitals can increase their local customary inpatient fees by more than 200% and be paid under this new rule and I have seen evidence of this at one Demo hospital already that openly advertises higher Demo prices and lower prices for everyone else.

Another policy reversal remains secret as TMA/DHA has refused to clarify the policy for the last year. In March 2013 a retiree came to me with two EOBs and a receipt for laboratory work done under the Demo. The receipt showed 7 specific lab procedures along with their prices. One EOB also showed the same 7 lab procedures and the same prices but showed the claim had been denied as a duplicate claim; but no paid EOB ever appeared. The second EOB showed a claim for 7 "Other and Unspecified Office Visits", all on the same day as the lab procedures and a total amount billed that was identical to the total cost of the 7 lab tests. The full amount was allowed for payment. This appeared to be either fraud on the part of the hospital or WPS. If the claim had been processed using the CMAC a significant portion of the billed amounts would have been disallowed and the beneficiary would have been due a refund on their co-pay. We submitted an appeal on behalf of the beneficiary and about two months later a response was received claiming the claim had been properly paid under current policy. We followed that up with a call to WPS and was told that they had been wrongly processing claims for the previous five years and should have been paying billed charges for all hospital services provided on an outpatient basis. We were also told that all claims that had been improperly processed would be reprocessed under the change.

At that point we tried to obtain confirmation from TMA/DHA on this policy and assurances that five years' worth of claims would be reprocessed. After many months and multiple reminders we finally received confirmation that this was true. But we were also told that they saw no reason to reprocess claims as the payments would not be significantly different; I know that was not true since I previously had similar claims underpaid by close to 40% under the old process. I also was provided an example of a Demo provider who was paid at billed charges for an MRI and at more than double the CMAC rates. Further they claimed there was no reason to notify beneficiaries of this as it was not really a change to policy; just a mistake.

Within days of receiving this information I had a claim for laboratory work processed and paid using the CMAC in an obvious violation of what TMA/DHA had just confirmed. My multiple inquires to WPS eventually resulted in a partial reversal of the policy saying that laboratory and radiology hospital claims were processed under the CMAC and instead of billed charges as they previously claimed and now in violation of what TMA/DHA told me. However, if this was true than I had evidence that they had paid multiple claims for these services to Demo providers at billed charges in violation of what now appeared to be another change.

I went back to TMA/DHA asking for a clarification of the policy in light of what WPS had just said and done. I also provided examples of claims that were significantly underpaid under the old process asking for reconsideration of relooking claims. It took ten months to get the first response and it has only been four months since I asked for the clarification and reconsideration so it may well be another six months before I get an answer. In the meantime we have no idea what is and what is not the real policy.

Bottom line it is clear that the Demo is going to cost both the taxpayer and beneficiaries a lot more money in higher fees negotiated by the contractor.

There are many other problems that appeared when the Demo was brought on line and to many to cover here; they may be addressed with examples in a later book. It should be obvious to most that TMA/DHA failed to develop a well thought out plan that considered the local health care industry standards and then turned their contractor loose to pretty much do as they pleased including lying to TMA/DHA about policies and practices they implemented. Because the contractor is paid millions to implement and manage this Demo, they have a vested interest in keeping it going at all costs, as with most companies the bottom line rules. For the government to allow a contractor and in particular a contractor with their history in the Philippines, to operate independently with nobody on the ground to observe the process and consequences seems to show how little concern TMA/DHA has for beneficiaries in the Philippines and the tax payer who will share in paying the bill. Failure to investigate allegations against the contractor and instead taking their word without question against beneficiaries also seems to show even less concern for beneficiaries and the taxpayer.

This also appears to be a violation of The Consumer Act of the Philippines, Republic Act No. 7394.

End Result

The end result of all of these actions has been to severely reduce access to care while increasing beneficiary cost significantly and TMA/DHA even admitted this in the *DODIG report 2014-052*[lvi], also addressed earlier. While the DODIG said TMA/DHA failed to provide proof of this I think I have done that throughout this book.

Access to care is so bad in the Philippines compared to anywhere else in the world, a number of retirees who opted to cancel Medicare Part B, which also removes them from TRICARE. They feel that they will not be reimbursed by TRICARE and can't use Medicare here so can better use the money to fund their own care.

To try to make it abundantly clear just how bad it is and to use the latest data, I will do a down and dirty comparison that, while understating the expected per capita cost in the Philippines still shows a huge chasm between what should be paid and what is and much worse than the previous comparison addressed earlier.

In the TRICARE *Fiscal Year 2013 Report to Congress*[lvii] TMA/DHA reported on page 90 of the report that the average under 65 retiree/survivor and family member on Standard/Extra utilized $8,515 of health care with $7,476 paid by TRICARE per beneficiary. On page 93 of the report the average 65 and over retiree/survivor and family member on Standard/Extra utilized $15,664 of which TRICARE and Medicare paid $15,175 per beneficiary; TRICARE Overseas covers what Medicare would pay in the states.

The DODIG in Report 2014-052 states that in 2012, $3,610,817 was spent by TRICARE on beneficiary medical care in the Philippines.

Using the DOD Actuary report of retirees and survivors in the Philippines in 2012 and a factor of 1.69 to calculate family members there would have been 11,782 TRICARE beneficiaries in 2012.

The TMA/DHA says the cost of care in the Philippines is 54% of what it costs in the U.S. except that the cost of pharmaceuticals, laboratory and radiology is at 100% and higher cost inpatient care generally involving open heart surgery and cancer treatments are closer to 80% of the cost in the U.S. as well; mostly due to high cost medical supplies.

If we forget the higher cost areas and assume everything costs 54% of what it costs in the states. And if we assume that no Philippines beneficiary is 65 or over[31] and take 54% of $7,476 we find it comes to $4,037. But in 2012 they spent $306 per beneficiary in the Philippines.

That works out to 7.6%, ($306 ÷ $4,037) of what is spent on under 65 beneficiaries and a clear indicator that what TMA/DHA told the DODIG is true. Further the information I provided for these calculations are available to anyone on the internet including TMA/DHA and the DODIG.

If one was to consider the relative higher cost of care by calculating the percentage that applies to ancillary costs and also used the percentages of 65 and over beneficiaries per the DOD Actuary the percentage would drop considerably and be closer to 4% or less of what would be expected.

Even if you don't consider those points, it should be clear that even at 7.6% something is dramatically wrong and it should be clear that TMA/DHA and the DODIG are looking the other way to protect their agendas.

Alternatives Available to TMA/DHA to Provide an Equal Benefit in the Philippines

The one policy change they agreed to implement but made little effort to do was a contracted local HMO/PPO.[32] There was a halfhearted attempt to solicit input for an extremely short period of time with essentially no direction on what they wanted and then it was dropped. In addition the solicitation was directed towards U.S. companies rather than towards those in the Philippines that could provide the expected service. So in reality they made no attempt to implement what Mr. Boucek indicated in his *article*[lviii] that they agreed to implement; that being a partnership with a local Philippine HMO/PPO which would have a functional network of approved providers operating under a reasonable cost schedule.

In 2009 and after submitting written justification and having lengthy conversations with MG Granger, who was the Deputy

---

[31] The DOD Actuary data for 2012 indicates that 52% of retirees are 65 and over while 72% of survivors are 65 and over.

[32] Generally what is called an HMO in the Philippines more closely resembles a PPO in the U.S.

80

Director of TMA at the time, he agreed that a locally contracted HMO/PPO would be a good solution to both the fraud issues and developing access to care hindrances caused by other policy changes. His goal was to implement it here and then evaluate the results for possible porting to other countries. However he retired before he was able to accomplish his objective. His attempt to visit the Philippines in 2009 to consult with beneficiaries concerning their concerns and issues was also denied for reasons that were never made clear to me.

A few years ago the Military Health System (MHS) solicited recommendations from industry and individuals for recommendations on how to reduce TRICARE cost. I took the initiative to prepare a study, based on the recommendation for using a local HMO/PPO. Using my background it health care administration and knowledge of the local health care industry I interviewed local medical insurance providers and obtained general estimates of cost and ability to provide a benefit that would match the TRICARE benefit. I submitted the study through the MHS internet portal that was soliciting recommendations. While I received an automated response indicating it was received, no further interest was apparently generated.

Bottom line

No place else in the world has this combination of policies been put into place and implemented and without adequate understanding of the full ramifications of the policies in relation to the local health care industry or adequate training of beneficiaries or monitoring of contractors. Unless someone in a position of authority decides to take action or the media decides to bring this suffering to the light of day, there will eventually be virtually no TRICARE benefit in the Philippines and many will suffer and die as a result.

This should also be a warning to beneficiaries living in other countries such as Japan, South Korea, the United Kingdom, Bahrain, Turkey and probably others countries. This book is an outline of the plans the DODIG and TMA/DHA have in mind for you, as well as the long term affects. The DODIG in Report 2014-052 makes that pretty clear!

I encourage you to contact me at ForgottenFewPI@gmail.com if you have questions, examples of how we are treated overseas or evidence of fraud on the part of the contractors.

ⁱ http://actuary.defense.gov/

ⁱⁱ http://www.highbeam.com/doc/1P1-79264815.html

ⁱⁱⁱ https://dl.dropboxusercontent.com/u/14030086/NewsLetter/Nov   Update/HVC Locations_3.pdf

^{iv} https://dl.dropboxusercontent.com/u/14030086/ArticleByBoucek-1.pdf

^v https://dl.dropboxusercontent.com/u/14030086/ArticleByBoucek-1.pdf

^{vi} D:\Jim's Documents\DOC\Congressional Issues\Barber\Question for DHA Armed Svc Committee Feb 14\D-2011-107

^{vii} https://dl.dropboxusercontent.com/u/14030086/Book/Please find below the answer from Douglas Robb.pdf

^{viii} https://dl.dropboxusercontent.com/u/14030086/DODIG Reports/11-107.pdf

^{ix} http://www.dodig.mil/pubs/documents/D-2011-107.pdf

^x https://dl.dropboxusercontent.com/u/14030086/Book/Please find below the answer from Douglas Robb.pdf

^{xi} http://www.youtube.com/watch?v=BOQAVfgf7yQ

^{xii} http://us4.campaign-archive1.com/?u=1559742f080d1da5be82951cf&id=b47d3078cb

^{xiii} http://data.worldbank.org/indicator/FP.CPI.TOTL.ZG

^{xiv} https://dl.dropboxusercontent.com/u/14030086/Receipts/8JanReceipt.pdf

^{xv} https://dl.dropboxusercontent.com/u/14030086/Book/Kyl %28H%29 Response_2.pdf

^{xvi} https://dl.dropboxusercontent.com/u/14030086/Book/Request for assistance in coding claims.pdf

^{xvii} https://dl.dropboxusercontent.com/u/14030086/Book/Phy Itemized.PDF

^{xviii} https://dl.dropboxusercontent.com/u/14030086/Book/CPTDenial.pdf

^{xix} https://dl.dropboxusercontent.com/u/14030086/Book/Provider Claim Breakout Letters.pdf

^{xx} https://dl.dropboxusercontent.com/u/14030086/Analysis/Analysis of Fiscal Year 2009 Philippine TRICARE Claims Data.pdf

^{xxi} https://dl.dropboxusercontent.com/u/14030086/ClosedNetwork/Surveys/Philippine TRICARE Survey Mar 13 wo Names.pdf

^{xxii} http://www.dodig.mil/pubs/documents/DODIG-2014-052.pdf

^{xxiii} http://www.gpo.gov/fdsys/pkg/GAOREPORTS-T-HEHS-00-138/html/GAOREPORTS-T-HEHS-00-138.htm

^{xxiv} https://dl.dropboxusercontent.com/u/14030086/Book/Kyl2011Response.pdf

^{xxv} https://dl.dropboxusercontent.com/u/14030086/ProgramIntegrity.ppt

^{xxvi} https://dl.dropboxusercontent.com/u/14030086/Analysis/Analysis of Fiscal Year 2009 Philippine TRICARE Claims Data.pdf

^{xxvii} https://dl.dropboxusercontent.com/u/14030086/Congress/The Elimination of the TRICARE Medical Benefit for Military Retirees in the PhilippinesRevised.pdf

^{xxviii} https://dl.dropboxusercontent.com/u/14030086/ArticleByBoucek-1.pdf

^{xxix} https://www.federalregister.gov/articles/2011/09/28/2011-24901/tricare-demonstration-project-for-the-philippines

^{xxx} http://www.stripes.com/news/tricare-scrapping-troubled-system-in-philippines-to-address-fraud-military-retiree-care-1.161832

^{xxxi} http://actuary.defense.gov/

^{xxxii} https://dl.dropboxusercontent.com/u/14030086/Book/Claims Graph.pdf

^{xxxiii} http://www.consumerreports.org/cro/magazine/2012/07/that-ct-scan-costs-how-much/index.htm

^{xxxiv} http://data.worldbank.org/indicator/FP.CPI.TOTL.ZG

^{xxxv} http://db.tt/DeZBrbts

xxxvi   http://www.stripes.com/news/pacific/philippines/retirees-still-to-face-upfront-medical-payments-in-philippines-1.197918

xxxvii   http://www.stripes.com/news/two-key-hospitals-quit-tricare-pilot-project-for-retirees-in-philippines-1.249930#tabs_7_8971_1381436415_1170486_tab4

xxxviii   http://www.stripes.com/news/dha-hopes-billing-fix-will-bring-back-philippine-hospitals-that-quit-pilot-project-1.251100

xxxix https://dl.dropboxusercontent.com/u/14030086/NewsLetter/Nov Update/Philippine Population Graphics.pdf

xl   https://dl.dropboxusercontent.com/u/14030086/NewsLetter/Nov Update/Philippine Population Graphics.pdf

xli http://actuary.defense.gov/

xlii   https://dl.dropboxusercontent.com/u/14030086/ClosedNetwork/Surveys/Philippine TRICARE Survey Mar 13 wo Names.pdf

xliii https://dl.dropboxusercontent.com/u/14030086/NewsLetter/Nov Update/How Do They Do It.pdf

xliv   https://dl.dropboxusercontent.com/u/14030086/NewsLetter/Nov Update/HVC Map.pdf

xlv   https://dl.dropboxusercontent.com/u/14030086/NewsLetter/Nov Update/HVC Map.pdf

xlvi https://dl.dropboxusercontent.com/u/14030086/NewsLetter/Nov Update/TRICARE Beneficiary Population Distribution Information.pdf

xlvii   https://www.federalregister.gov/articles/2011/09/28/2011-24901/tricare-demonstration-project-for-the-philippines

xlviii https://dl.dropboxusercontent.com/u/14030086/ClosedNetwork/C24S4.pdf

xlix http://youtu.be/BOQAVfgf7yQ

l http://www.tricare.mil/patientrights

li http://www.dtic.mil/whs/directives/corres/pdf/600014p.pdf

lii http://www.tricare.mil/patientrights

liii   http://www.washingtonpost.com/wp-dyn/content/graphic/2006/04/07/GR2006040700882.html

liv https://dl.dropboxusercontent.com/u/14030086/Book/Policy Reversal Evidence.pdf

lv https://dl.dropboxusercontent.com/u/14030086/Book/Policy Reversal Evidence.pdf

lvi http://www.dodig.mil/pubs/documents/DODIG-2014-052.pdf

lvii   http://www.health.mil/Reference-Center/Reports/2013/02/28/Evaluation-of-the-TRICARE-Program-Fiscal-Year-2013-Report-to-Congress

lviii https://dl.dropboxusercontent.com/u/14030086/ArticleByBoucek-1.pdf

www.ingramcontent.com/pod-product-compliance
Lightning Source LLC
Chambersburg PA
CBHW021343290326
41933CB00037B/542